Being a

BLESSING

והיה ברכה

54 Ways You Can Help People Living with AIDS

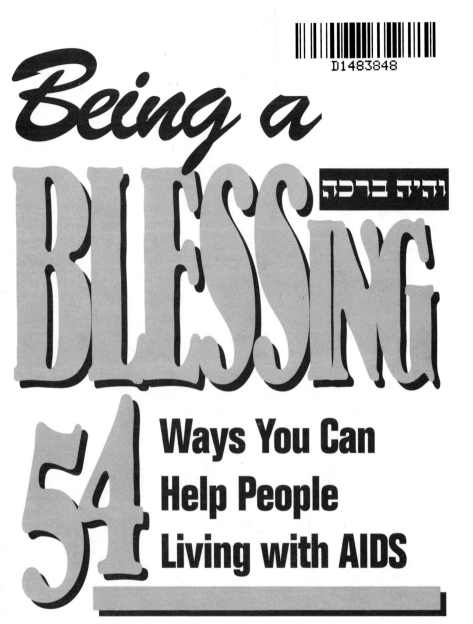

Rabbi Harris R. Goldstein

with a foreword by Rabbi Daniel H. Freelander

Library of Congress Cataloging-in-Publication Data
Goldstein, Harris R., 1955-
    Being A Blessing : 54 ways you can help people living with AIDS /
Harris R. Goldstein.
        p.   cm.
    Includes bibliographical references and index.
    ISBN 1-881283-08-9 : $12.95
    1. AIDS (Disease)—Patients—Care. 2. AIDS (Disease)—Patients—Services for.
3. AIDS (Disease)—Religous aspects—Judaism.
    RC607.A26G56   1994
    362.1969792—dc20   94-3620
                                                                CIP

Copyright © 1994 Rabbi Harris R. Goldstein

ISBN # 0-831283-08-9

Published by Alef Design Group

Alef Design Group
4423 Fruitland Avenue
Los Angeles, California 90058
(213) 582-1200

Dedicated:

in memory of

Melvin Lloyd Rosen	Scott Friedland
Richard Laks	Dr. Scott Billig
Michael Olowacz	Jack Bier
Katlyn Wolf	Robert Cooper
Colleen Wolf	David Velez
Louis Perez	Michael Callen
Dr. Eliot Bernstein	

May their memory continue to be a blessing for all whose lives they've touched;

In honor of Vivian Torres, Anna Chaljub, Dr. Elliot Gold, John Henri, Francis Maloney, James Buckrham, Joel Cabrera, Geraldine Hill, Teri Pfaeffle and all of the other people who are fighting AIDS with their hearts, minds and bodies;

In honor of, and thanks to, all of the people who make a difference in the lives of people living with AIDS;

To J.B., whose love and friendship, guidance and support have made my work possible.

*A*cknowledgments:

Rabbi J.B. Sacks provided tremendous resources, encouragement, enthusiasm, energy and inspiration for this book. Many of the ways of helping people living with AIDS listed in this book are from J.B.'s suggestions and guidance. The Rev. Laura Lee Kent-Smith, Executive Director of the AIDS Interfaith Network of New Jersey, trained me in AIDS service delivery and in developing techniques for involvement of congregations in direct-service AIDS ministry. Gloria S. Rubin helped me and encouraged me in the process of writing this manuscript, and her suggestions helped make it much more reader-friendly. Rabbi Dr. Shohama Wiener, Executive Dean of the Academy for Jewish Religion, has served as my spiritual guide in the journey through life and death. This book was written in fulfillment of the requirements for the Senior Rabbinical Project at the Academy for Jewish Religion.

I would especially like to thank the many congregations, individuals and denominational groups with whom I worked in the development of direct-service AIDS Mitzvah Programs and AIDS prevention educational programs.

Table of Contents

Foreword 7
Introduction 10
Starfish Story 15

Section 1: *Talmud Torah*...17
1. Learn Basic AIDS Information (AIDS 101) 19
2. How You Can and Cannot be Infected with HIV 20
3. Understand the Connection Between Mind and Body 22
4. What Do People Living with AIDS Need from People of Faith? 25
5. Learn How Language Has an Impact on the Lives of People Living with AIDS. 26
6. Understand What It Means to be Created in the Image of God.................28
7. Become Familiar with, Help Others Understand "People with AIDS Bill of Rights" ...31
8. Understand How to Help the "System" 33
9. Understand the Need for Confidentiality..35

Section 2: *Pikuach Nefesh*–Saving Life/Self-Protection 37
10. Learn about Risk and Abstinence 39
11. Develop an AIDS Prevention Educational Program for Teenagers. 42
12. Help Combat the Myths, Misinformation, and Prejudice Associated with AIDS.........50
13. Develop an AIDS Resource Center..52

Section 3: *Bikkur Holim*–Visiting the Sick 53
14. When You Visit. 55
15. Bring Food to Someone who is Homebound/in the hospital..................60
16. Bring Something to Do..61
17. Make Phone Calls to People Living with AIDS. 62
18. Develop a Phone Team for Daily Conversations with People Living with AIDS.........63
19. Visit and Provide Breaks for Primary Caretakers 64
20. Cards, Flowers, Plants, Things to Brighten a Bleak Room. 66
21. Make Warm, Fuzzy Items for People Living with AIDS...........................67
22. Hold Drives to Collect Books, Tapes and Games 68
23. Provide Transportation. 70
24. Develop a Bikur Holim (Visiting the Sick) Committee............................71
25. Prepare Holiday and Sabbath Gift Baskets 72

Section 4: *Shituf B'tsaar*–Alleviating Another's Pain................................73
26. Host a Dinner for People Living with AIDS, Families/Loved Ones, Friends. 75
27. Pray/Meditate with People Living with AIDS. 78
28. Arrange for Services of Comfort and Hope. 85

5

29. Incorporate Prayers for People Living with AIDS into Congregational Services and Events. 90
30. Become a Funding Partner of an AIDS Service Provider. 91
    Collecting Things for People Living with AIDS...93
31. Collect Food for People Living with AIDS...95
32. Collect Over-the-Counter Medications, Personal Hygiene Products. 97
33. Collect Household Supplies for People Living with AIDS. 99
34. Collect Clothing for People Living with AIDS. 100
35. Develop a Plan for Distribution of the Supplies Collected in 31–34 Above. 103
36. Think About the Things You or Your Company Uses or Makes. 105
37. Visit a Display of the AIDS Memorial Quilt, or Arrange for a Display..106
38. Create a Panel for the Quilt..108
39. Say Kaddish for People Who Have Died of AIDS. 110
40. Develop a Transportation System for People Living with AIDS..111
41. Invite People Living with AIDS to Holiday and Shabbat Events 113
42. Take Care of a Child of a Person Living with AIDS..114

Section 5: *Tikkun Olam*—Make the World a Better Place 116
43. Arrange to Deliver Hot Meals to Homebound People Living with AIDS 119
44. Cook Special Meals for People Living with AIDS in Group Homes...121
45. Develop an Unrestricted Fund for Emergencies..123
46. Provide Special Programs for Professional Caregivers. 125
47. Provide Space for AIDS Service Providers to Hold Support Group Meetings or Leadership Meetings...128
48. Help Facilitate Support Groups for Unmet Needs 129
49. Lead Letter-Writing Campaigns to Politicians. 133
50. Give of YourselfYour Own Talents and Professional Abilities. 134
51. Give Money. 135
52. Include Funds for People Living with AIDS in Your Celebrations...137
53. Make Holidays More Spiritually Meaningful with Special Donations. 139
54. Stand Up for Civil Rights of People Living with AIDS...140
Final Thoughts..141

AIDS Glossary...143
Glossary of Hebrew Terms 146
Resource Directory 149
    Directories..149
    Hotlines..150
    Treatment Information and Newsletters 150
    Agencies and Services 151
    Books on Surviving AIDS...154

I t has been said that a society's values are most accurately reflected in the way it responds to serious disease. And disease on an epidemic scale brings to the fore all our deepest fears—both rational and irrational—and often renders us incapable of responding in useful or meaningful ways. We act in ways that help few, if any, of those who suffer:

We choose to ignore the plague, saying that the media is exaggerating its spread and overplaying its importance or danger.

We choose to assume ourselves immune, believing that only "others" will be affected. We do, after all, live in the clean, safe suburbs, surrounded by neighbors just like us.

We believe that we are above it all, that due to upbringing, education or personal religious practice, we and our families will be spared the plague's ravages.

We express anger at those who bring the disease into our midst, and seek to isolate them, and hence its further spread.

We keep our children from knowing anything about its reality, lest they become scared or worried.

We view the inexplicable plague as divine retribution against immoral behavior.

This has been humanity's normative response to those diseases whose sources and cures evade us; witness society's less-than-humane initial reaction to Leprosy, to the Black Plague, etc.

We Americans have shown similar tendencies to distance ourselves from traumatic catastrophes around the world. We just don't take note of the urgency of a crisis until irreparable damage has been done. We read of the genocide in Bosnia and Rwanda. We view pictures of thousands starving-and we are moved, but not quite enough to do anything about it.

We've come to accept the reality of homelessness and hunger in our cities and towns, asserting that the problem is beyond our ability to help. We allow ourselves to perceive the problem to be beyond our capabilities to solve. And because we, as individuals, cannot fathom a solution, we ignore the problem altogether, as though it did not exist.

Good people throughout history have responded to Anti-Semitism in a similar manner. The government, or the Klan, or the Skinheads, etc. might be acting in ways that are abhorrent, but speaking out against injustice or discrimination might get one in trouble. One might lose social status if aligned with society's "others." And so, as with disease, we render the problem "unhandleable," and hope that it will go away and not become worse.

But have we learned nothing from Jewish history? It is the "righteous Gentiles" who spoke out on our behalf whom we now revere. It is visionary leaders who saw the need to mobilize society's resources to fight diseases or famines or injustice whom we now credit with bettering this world. Our Biblical prophets taught our people this. Our sacrifices were meaningless without our personal efforts to be God's partners in implementing the ethics of our tradition in this world.

So it is with AIDS. We can easily distance ourselves, denying its impact on our lives. We keep our basic information on safe sexual practices from our children, hoping they will instinctively know never to engage in unprotected sex. We can hold debates on universal health insurance as though we or our children will never lose our coverage.

I, too, chose to ignore the reality of AIDS in its early days. And I don't know if I would have been shaken out of my comfortable fantasy if AIDS had not appeared on our family's doorstep in 1985.

For two excruciating years I watched as AIDS ravaged my brother's body, mind and emotions. I watched the pain of my parents' struggling against all odds to save their son. I watched the indifference of the Jewish community to the fact that many AIDS patients were Jews. "This is not a Jewish issue," they would say, "let's not make it into one." But ultimately, my own defenses against dealing with uncomfortable realities melted as my brother put a human face on AIDS.

Unfortunately, my understanding of the danger of inaction came too late for me to make a real difference in my brother's life. Since his death in 1987, I have come to appreciate the importance of those small grassroots we can each make to address the injustice and misinformation that accompanies diseases that are beyond our control.

The religious community has a unique role to play in combating AIDS. No effort is too small to have meaning in the continuing battle against the disease. Our children and our neighbors need role models. They need us to do those small things that when added together may ultimately make a difference. They need us to model appropriate behaviors of caring and responsibility towards others. They need us not to be afraid to act.

Harris Goldstein's volume instructs us on how we can become those role models. We can't eradicate AIDS. We can't heal all those who are sick. We can't eliminate all the human pain AIDS has caused. But we can play our small role in helping to eradicate misinformation and irrational fears, easing the suffering of those who live with HIV/AIDS and bringing comfort and support to the thousands who continue to be touched by this plague.

The ultimate measure of our Jewish community's values will be our ability to rise above personal self interests and behave towards others as someday we may need them to behave towards us.

Lo BaShamayim Hi. The solutions to AIDS and hurtful human behaviors are not in heaven. They are in our hearts, our mouths, our minds and our hands.

Daniel Hillel Freelander
Director of Programs, UAHC
Av, 5754

Introduction

I became involved in the struggle to help people living with AIDS because I felt I had put off involvement for too long. I was working at the Jewish Federation of North Jersey as the Campaign Director, raising funds to help Jews all over the world and in the local Jewish community. But I felt very disconnected from the people who were benefiting from my work, and though I continue to believe in the work of the Federations and United Jewish Appeal, I kept feeling that we were missing an important segment of the Jewish community in need. I was attending services at Congregation Beth Simchat Torah in New York (the world's largest synagogue serving the gay and lesbian community), and every week, it seemed, we were saying kaddish (the prayer for the dead) for another member who had died of AIDS that week. This, in a congregation where the average age is probably under 40 years.

The Jewish communal response to AIDS has been minimal. When I talk to rabbis, they tell me no one in their congregations is affected; no one has come to them to perform a funeral, to visit the sick, or to be a source of support or comfort for the families. Young people whom they have buried have died of other causes.

Yet, whenever I or my colleagues speak at a Jewish communal function, we are always approached by people who need to share their grief, their concern, and their fears. They don't go to their own rabbis because they do not yet see the rabbis as receptive to AIDS. They don't come to the very people who could provide the spiritual comfort they need and deserve.

The funeral homes are busy, but who is officiating at the funerals? More importantly, where are the Jewish communities before the funerals? We, as a Jewish community, must respond to this epidemic. We are not doing nearly enough by just burying the dead.

I must respond to this epidemic. It took me a long time to realize that I was not doing enough. I came to that realization last July, on my thirty-sixth birthday. A non-Jewish friend of mine had made a small dinner party for me. He couldn't understand why the number 36, double _ḥai_, was so important to me. At dinner, after we talked about the concept of _ḥai_, the conversation turned to AIDS: who died last week, who was going to die this week, and whose memorial service was being announced. An odd conversation, but all too typical these days. One of the people at dinner asked, "Are we doing enough?" Each of us was visiting the sick, attending the funerals, comforting the survivors.

Elana said that she thought that when we look back at this epidemic, 15 years after it is over, we will be just like the Germans after the Holocaust who didn't really know what was going on until it was too late. They didn't do enough because they didn't know. We, on the other hand, do know, and are therefore doing plenty.

I went wild. First, I wasn't about to allow history to be rewritten so easily. The Germans knew exactly what was happening to the Jews and made it happen. Secondly, I knew I was not doing enough. I left that dinner knowing that I was not doing enough, whatever "enough" is, and that not doing enough was precisely what I found most confusing about my parents' generation during the Holocaust. I realized that in many ways AIDS is a holocaust taking place today. Maybe it's not inspired by a madman, but there are indeed many villains in this case.

At Congregation Beth Simchat Torah, the congregation has accepted responsibility for a Holocaust Torah from Czechoslovakia. They have built a beautiful memorial case to honor it and have made a new home for a Torah from a congregation which will never be redeemed. Next to this Torah and the Holocaust memorial is the shul's memorial wall. This memorial is filling and being expanded at a horrific rate with the names of people whose lives have been cut short, who should not be dying, whose deaths we cannot accept or comprehend.

A reminder and memorial of one holocaust in a time of another. It should remind all of us to ask the same questions I demanded of my parents. Are we doing enough?

The AIDS epidemic is, at times, overwhelming. So many people are directly affected. So much needs to be done to prevent the continued spread, and to care for the needs of people living with AIDS. We can't change the world. But we can touch individuals and make a difference in each of their lives.

Many people ask me why a disease is a Jewish, or religious, issue. After all, we don't have people coming and talking about Jewish responsibility for heart disease, or cancer, or muscular dystrophy. But we also do not, as a society, abandon and disconnect from people with these ailments. In many ways, AIDS is a test for all of us, to see if we really believe in what we say about *tikkun olam* (fixing the world) or what we say about caring for the ill and the downtrodden, or what we think is doing the right thing by people. AIDS is not a medical issue for us, it is an issue of human dignity, decency, value and honor.

Caring for people with AIDS is not just caring for people suffering from a disease; it's really about making personal connections with people who are disconnected from society. Because too many people, for too long, have treated people with AIDS like lepers.

There is another reason that we, as Jews, or as people of faith, must get involved in this struggle: AIDS is contagious and can be prevented. We have a sacred obligation to preserve life. If people are provided with proper education, AIDS/HIV can be prevented. But our school systems are not doing an adequate job of prevention education. AIDS/HIV is not a disease that affects a group of people at risk. It is a threat to all people who engage in unsafe sexual relations.

Our teenagers are not getting that message, and there is an explosion of AIDS/HIV in heterosexual teenagers, women, and children. We delude ourselves into thinking that this disease affects just a few definable groups of people. Once the first wave is dead, will we continue to blame the victims?

When it seemed it was a disease of only gay people and Haitians, everyone else was immune. When it became a disease that affected IV drug users, we didn't have to worry, since they were dispensable anyway. Now that we know that it effects everyone, and that millions of people from all walks of life are going to be killed by this disease, the miseducation of the past few years will continue to take its toll.

Kids always think of themselves as immortal, or that they are not touched by death. From what they have heard, if they are not homosexual and do not shoot up drugs, they can do what they want. I spoke with an 18-year-old who is active sexually with men and women. When I asked him if he uses a condom, he said he did when he was with men. But he doesn't when he is with his girlfriend, since she thinks he's monogamous and certainly doesn't know he's also having intercourse with other men. He's not atypical. Today, one in every 300 students at Rutgers University is HIV-positive. It doesn't take a lot of imagination to see what that means for our future.

But we can help put an end to this nightmare. To be able to answer the question "Are we doing enough?" we have to do three things: institute AIDS prevention education in our high schools and junior high schools; begin reaching out to people with AIDS and working with them to make their lives easier; and begin public advocacy on behalf of people living with AIDS and to find a cure. All of these actions are necessary, all demand personal involvement, and none can be done for us by others.

Lives are at stake. We cannot leave it up to the public schools, because they are simply not effective in teaching about AIDS. For instance, when we heard an AIDS prevention lesson recently, the teacher kept talking about "intimate contact" as the way that AIDS/HIV is spread. Those two words were never defined. It leaves an awful lot to the imagination.

We also cannot leave responsibility for people living with AIDS to the government. It has already proven miserably inadequate to the task. Living with AIDS/HIV can be so difficult. Our medical system is ill equipped to meet the needs of people with AIDS. And our social systems don't even approach their needs. If you are tested, as we recommend to everyone, and your results are positive for the HIV antibodies, you can move very quickly to abject poverty.

AIDS is different. For too long the bigots of the religious communities were most vocal when it came to responding to AIDS. In the name of

God, they said that this disease was divine retribution for the sins of the "perverts," who got what they deserved. Our government, on the other hand, remained silent when vigorous response was necessary, precisely because the people most affected by AIDS were gay men and intravenous drug users. In other words, people living with AIDS were expendable. During the first 8 years of the AIDS crisis, the president of the United States, Ronald Reagan, never once mentioned the word AIDS. His successor, George Bush, did little more.

The role of religion in our lives is, in a large part, to make the world a better place, to help people in need, to correct injustice, to make us better human beings. These values are shared by Jews and Christians alike. It is precisely because of the bigotry, the misinformation, and the continued lack of response of our government that religious groups have to step in and say, "This is not how we treat our fellow human beings." It is precisely the role of people of faith to put their faith into action when, in the name of God, wrongs have been done, when the secular response fails us. When people who are ill are considered to be unworthy of care, when illness is seen as judgment, when people are abandoned, intentionally hurt, or emotionally battered because they have a virus, it is up to communities of faith to respond by leading the way to fairness and justice.

As I began talking in the suburban Jewish and non-Jewish communities, it became obvious how much need there is out there. Outside New York City, AIDS services—especially those programs which are not medically based—are virtually nonexistent. With the exception of the AIDS Interfaith Network of New Jersey, there are no programs involving substantial numbers of volunteers from suburban communities in the day-to-day life and needs of people living with AIDS in New Jersey. For the most part, I found people who were ready and willing, and often able, to make a meaningful impact on the crisis with their funds, their efforts, and their goodwill. As I spoke at more congregations (both Jewish and non-Jewish), I found a tremendous willingness to drop the bigotry surrounding the crisis, and to respond as people of faith are supposed to in a crisis: with care, compassion and hard work. While I did hear from one rabbi that he was unwilling to participate in helping "perverts and sinners," the vast majority of religious leaders with whom I met needed only to be pointed in the right direction and given some guidance and advice.

In addition to receptive clergy, I also met many people who wanted to become personally involved, or to involve their congregations, but did not know how to go about it. Short of finding people in hospitals or calling clinics, they were unsure as to how to help people living with AIDS directly. This book is intended as an answer to their questions, and the questions of clergy, as to how they can become more actively involved in the struggle to bring dignity, spiritual healing, hope and love to people who continue to be rejected by many people in our society.

This book is based on five Jewish values and how they apply to the AIDS epidemic. Each value is defined at the beginning of its section, and examples are cited from biblical and/or rabbinic sources as to the meaning of each value. Each section of this book is intended to suggest ways for individuals, clergy, groups and congregations to provide direct services and support services for people living with AIDS, bringing the value into reality.

Starfish Story

As an old man walked down the beach one day, he saw a child picking something up from the sand and throwing it into the sea. The old man asked the child, "What are you doing?" "Chucking starfish," the child replied. "Why?" asked the old man. "The starfish washed ashore in the high tide. If they stay on the beach, they will dry out and die, so I'm chucking them back into the ocean." The old man looked at the child and at the beach and said, "There are hundreds of starfish on this beach. How can what you're doing make any difference?"

The child bent down, picked up another starfish, pointed to it, and said, "It makes a difference to this one," and he threw it into the sea.

The rabbis teach in *Pirkei Avot* (2:15) that the task is hard and time is short. It's not up to you to finish the job, but neither are you exempt from getting it started.

What we are doing, in living with and assisting people living with AIDS, is chucking starfish. We may not be able to save the life of every person living with AIDS, we may not be able to bring hope and peace to all of them, but for the people whose lives we touch, what we do makes a real and meaningful difference. We may not be able to touch all of the lives which are devastated by AIDS, but if each of us takes responsibility for chucking just a few starfish during our lifetimes, we will collectively have made a real difference for a lot of people.

This book is, in many ways, a guidebook for 54 ways to chuck starfish. 54 is three times _hai_ (18), which means three times life. In Hebrew, each letter has a numerical value. The letters which make up the word _hai_ (life) add up to 18. When you "chuck starfish," when you help people living with AIDS, three lives are touched. The life of the person being helped and your own life are obvious. You will be transformed by the good of your work, by the sacredness of your mission. After you see the impact of your deeds on someone else's life, your life will never be the same again. The people living with AIDS whom you help will likewise be transformed by your generosity and your understanding of your role in the world. You will show that not all people are bigots, that people of faith can take meaningful action to help people in need. The peace of mind and body you bring will save lives, save spirits and save souls.

The third life that is touched is less obvious. But when you help people living with AIDS, when you fulfill the _mitzvot_ (commandments) listed in this book, you bring the _Shekhinah_ (Divine Presence) to dwell among us, to participate in helping make the world a better place. The third symbolic life is that of the Divine Presence. God depends on us to do God's work, with our own hands, with our own hearts. Know that every interaction you have to help people living with AIDS, every conversation, every good deed, every meal or every event, is infused with the spirit of the _Shekhinah_, and that you are doing God's work with your own hands. God is the third partner of every lifesaving or life-enhancing step you take.

Thank you for joining in the task, for taking the steps. May your walk on this journey with people living with AIDS be blessed by the Divine Presence of God.

Section 1: Talmud Torah

Learn and teach: We are obligated to learn in order to understand what God expects of us. We are obligated to use our knowledge to help ourselves become better people, and to assist other people.

In the Book of Ecclesiastes, we read, "For as wisdom grows, vexation grows. To increase learning is to increase heartache." This seems to imply that we should stop learning, because who needs an increase in "vexation?" But as we learn, we become increasingly self-aware and aware of the other people in our world. If we are wise, we will value and appreciate the changes that happen to us as a result of our learning, even if those things we learn increase our levels of frustration, our need to take action, and our need to learn even more. The more we know, the more we realize how little we know, and how much work has yet to be done for us to gain wisdom.

Learning about AIDS is a good example. The more we know about AIDS, the more we come to understand what is yet unknown, what has yet to be done, and what we need to do personally in order to respond to our increasing "vexation". Learning about AIDS changes us forever in many ways. It can eliminate baseless fears, shake us from complacency, and help us better understand our roles in the greater order of things. Learning about AIDS is the first step in being able to respond to this epidemic.

Learning also demands teaching; the two go together. (Why suffer alone with increased heartache?) Part of wisdom is that it has to be shared. According to the Talmud (*Kiddushin* 29b-30a), a parent is obligated to teach a child Torah, a profession, and how to swim. The first two are obvious and have traditionally been implemented by Jews. Learning is something we have always valued. While at times secular learning has

17

taken precedence over Jewish learning, Jews have continued to teach their children to value and cherish their Judaism, often culminating with bar and bat mitzvah ceremonies. Secular learning has also been a high priority, and Jews have indeed heeded the commandment to teach their children a profession.

Teaching your child to swim, though, may not be so obvious. After all, people who don't particularly like to swim or don't live anywhere near water (or a pool) may not see the point. But it's not just to swim; the obligation of a parent is to teach a child how to preserve his or her life. Parents are obligated to teach their children to do whatever it is that they need to do in order to remain safe. In modern America, this would mean parents have to teach their children how to drive defensively and how to prepare for and respond to emergencies, like tornadoes or earthquakes. In addition to swimming, parents have to teach their children to survive in today's society, which means parents have to teach their children how *not* to get AIDS. While to many this may be an increase in heartache, it's nothing like losing a child to AIDS because of a lack of learning.

Judaism demands that we learn how to help other people, and this book is intended to enable people to learn, and to act based on what they have learned. As you learn Jewish values, you learn that Judaism has some very specific teachings that apply directly to the AIDS epidemic, and ultimately, that Judaism demands that you have a positive impact on the lives of people living with AIDS.

1. Learn Basic AIDS Information (AIDS 101)

The most important thing for you to know about AIDS is that you can't get it through casual contact. That means that you won't get AIDS from working with a person living with AIDS. You can be around people living with AIDS, you can have physical contact with people living with AIDS, you can breathe the air they breathe, you can eat the food they eat, you can drink the water they drink.

This book is not intended to be a scientifically complete treatise on AIDS or a medical textbook, but rather to provide information that will be helpful to you. If you would like more complete medical information, please contact your community's department of health or the Centers for Disease Control AIDS Hotline, 800-342-2437, Spanish Service SIDA, 800-344-7432, or TTY for hearing-impaired, 800-243-7889. The hotlines provide information, referrals and a nationwide database for treatment, testing sites, counseling, service organizations, referral for legal assistance and housing.

AIDS, acquired immunodeficiency syndrome, is not actually a disease, but rather a syndrome whereby a person's immune system is destroyed, leaving him/her open to infections and illness. Every person has an immune system that is supposed to keep one from getting ill. In a person living with AIDS, the immune system breaks down, so people living with AIDS get any number of illnesses their immune systems cannot ward off. People who have healthy immune systems don't get many of these illnesses. We still do not know what causes AIDS. The current theory holds that HIV (human immunodeficiency virus) attacks the immune system, causing its failure. There is no test for AIDS, but there is a test to detect whether the body has antibodies to HIV (meaning the body is trying to fight the virus).

2. How You Can and Cannot Be Infected with HIV

(Reprinted with permission from the *AIDS Prevention Guide: The Facts about HIV Infection and AIDS,* published by the Centers for Disease Control)

You can become infected with HIV in two main ways:

• Having sexual intercourse—vaginal, anal, or perhaps oral—with an infected person.

• Sharing drug needles or syringes with an infected person.

Also, women infected with HIV can pass the virus to their babies during pregnancy or during birth. In some cases they can also pass it on when breast-feeding. Some people have been infected by receiving blood transfusions, especially during the period prior to April, 1985, when careful screening and laboratory testing of the blood supply began.

How do you get HIV from sexual intercourse?

HIV can be spread through sexual intercourse, from male to female, female to male, or male to male. HIV may be in an infected person's blood, semen, or vaginal secretions. It is thought to enter the bloodstream through cuts or sores—some so small you don't know they're there—on tissue in the vagina, penis, or rectum and possibly the mouth.

Anal intercourse with an infected person is one of the ways HIV has been most frequently transmitted.

Since many infected people have no apparent symptoms of the condition, it's hard to be sure who is or who is not infected with HIV.

How do you get HIV from using needles?

Sharing needles or syringes, even once, is a very easy way to be infected with HIV and other germs. Sharing needles to inject IV drugs is the most dangerous form of needle sharing. Blood from an infected person can remain in or on a needle or syringe and then be transferred directly into the bloodstream of the next person who uses it.

Sharing other types of needles also may transmit HIV and other germs. These types of needles include those used to inject steroids and those used for tattooing or ear piercing.

If you plan to have your ears pierced or get a tattoo, make sure you go to a qualified technician who uses sterile equipment. Don't be shy about asking questions. Reputable technicians will explain the safety measures they follow.

What are ways by which you cannot get HIV and AIDS?

HIV infection doesn't just happen. You can't simply "catch" it like a cold or flu. Unlike cold or flu viruses, HIV is not spread through coughs or sneezes.

You won't get HIV through everyday contact with infected people at school, work, home, or anywhere else.

You won't get HIV from clothes, phones, or toilet seats. It can't be passed on by things like spoons, cups, or other objects that someone who is infected with the virus has used. You cannot get it from every-day contact with an infected person.

You won't get AIDS from a mosquito bite. The AIDS virus does not live in a mosquito, and it is not transmitted through a mosquito's salivary glands like other diseases such as malaria or yellow fever. You won't get it from bed bugs, lice, flies, or other insects, either.

You won't get HIV from sweat, tears, or sneezes. Even in the rare event that they contain any of the virus, they don't contain enough of the virus to infect you.

3. Understand the Connection Between Mind and Body

I s AIDS always fatal? How long will a person living with AIDS survive?

No one knows the answers to these questions. One thing we do know, though, is that when you tell people that they are going to die from one disease or another, they often cooperate with the prediction. At the outset of the discovery of AIDS, the medical community asserted that AIDS is 100% fatal. This overstatement of fatality may have been necessary to get research funds and to establish health policies, but there was neither scientific nor empirical data available at that time (or now) to prove that assertion. The prediction by certain people in the medical community that AIDS is 100% fatal may have contributed to fulfillment of that prophecy. Yes, a lot of people have died of complications from AIDS, from opportunistic infections that people living with AIDS get. Yet there are a lot of people whose immune systems are compromised, who have HIV antibodies and fewer than 200 "T" cells, and who are alive and well. There are a lot of people who have no symptoms of any opportunistic infections and are HIV positive. Unfortunately, not enough research has been done on these people to enable us to understand why some people survive AIDS.

Cancer used to be a fatal disease. We rarely look at cancer now as a completely untreatable killer, even though many people continue to die of cancers. People living with AIDS deserve the same optimistic outlook. We have only begun the process of understanding what happens to one's immune system when one has AIDS. We have only begun to explore therapies for treating the opportunistic infections associated with AIDS. Prophylaxis for opportunistic infections such as pneumocystis carinii pneumonia (PCP) has significantly reduced the death toll due to PCP. Unfortunately, other opportunistic infections have taken PCP's place. There will be therapies for them as well. Even though there will probably continue to be many deaths from AIDS, we will also be seeing many more people in the future living with the challenge of management of a range of opportunistic infections—people living with a chronic, not necessarily fatal, disease. (This all assumes the continued lack of a "cure". God willing, it should happen tomorrow, and we can all put our energies into other efforts. Nothing would make me happier than having my first book become completely obsolete!)

There has been some strong indication that mental attitude, physical fitness, proper diet, the avoidance of stress, and spiritual peacefulness can help in prolonging life and in the prevention of opportunistic infections. People who keep physically fit, take their vitamins, eat nutritious, well-balanced meals, get out of self-destructive behaviors, and make time every day for their own spiritual well-being tend to be the people who are "long-term" survivors. The Sunday *Parade* magazine on January 31, 1993 featured 6 long-term survivors, one of whom, George Melton, wrote a book on surviving AIDS, which I recommend highly. The article suggested that while all of the survivors were different, they all shared a sense of "spirituality and irreverence," "the grit, the pluck and courage to face up to almost anything," and a "sense of being chosen for an important mission." All look after their diets, keep physically fit, and have a positive outlook.

The connection between mind and body cannot be denied. Dr. Bernie Siegel, whose books *Love, Medicine and Miracles* and *Faith, Hope and Healing* are the definitive works on the connection between mind and body in cancer patients, asserts that people living with AIDS can also be "exceptional" patients by taking control of their medical care, gaining spiritual peacefulness, and having a positive outlook. Siegel makes it clear that people can have an impact on their destinies and the course of their diseases. Many people are able to find the inner peace that leads to healing of the spirit. Healing of the spirit is not synonymous with physical healing, though the two are intertwined. People who have found an inner peace may, however, progress through disease more calmly, with more confidence, and with significantly less pain, wherever the progression of the disease may lead. To help you fulfill this responsibility, I have attached a resource list on the topic of spirituality and healing for your future reference.

In the "AIDSFRONT" published bimonthly by the national gay magazine *The Advocate* (Issue 641, November 2, 1993), Dr. Martin Delaney, founding director of Project Inform, make the same point very succinctly:

> "In San Francisco, for example, the death rate from AIDS complications skyrocketed in the two months following the [Berlin] conference.[1] This had nothing to do with the effectiveness of therapy and everything to do with the power of thinking. False hopelessness remains the most virulent pathogen with AIDS, and conversely, hope remains the most potent therapy."

It is our job, as people of faith, to help people living with AIDS find the inner peace, the spirituality that is missing from so many lives. Times of need are precisely when people turn to their religious backgrounds for strength, renewal and hope. People living with AIDS should be able to turn to their clergy people and other members of their congregations for help in finding inner peace, understanding, and confidence in the ability of people to work wonders, of a right to hope and to have faith. We are responsible for bringing hope where there is despair.

---------- *Psalm 16:8,9,11* --

I am ever mindful of Adonai's presence; God is at my right hand; I shall never be shaken. So my heart rejoices, my whole being exults, and my body rests secure. For You will not abandon me. You will teach me the path of life. In Your presence is perfect joy; delights are ever in Your right hand.

---

[1] The 1993 Annual International AIDS Conference in Berlin was particularly depressing because there seemed to be no progress on finding either a cure or new treatments, and some evidence that the most common treatments, like AZT, were not working. The conference became a symbol of another year in a losing battle.

4. What Do People Living with AIDS Need from People of Faith?

PEOPLE LIVING WITH **AIDS** NEED support and care from people who are well. The most important thing people living with AIDS need from people who are well is assurance that though they face hard times and challenges ahead, they are not alone in the struggle. They can count on their families, their friends, their community, and their congregation for the spiritual, emotional and physical support they are going to need when times get rough.

PEOPLE LIVING WITH **AIDS** DON'T NEED pity or judgment—who does? People living with AIDS want to be treated just like anyone else. People living with AIDS have a chronic, life-threatening disease. The support and concern of those around them can go a long way in helping them face the challenges AIDS presents.

PEOPLE LIVING WITH **AIDS** NEED to know that you know that they are not "goners." People who are well can help people living with AIDS see that there is always hope, and they can draw strength from the resolve, faith and confidence of people who are well.

PEOPLE LIVING WITH **AIDS** NEED guarantees that they will not be hurt intentionally or unintentionally once they let people know that they are living with AIDS. To help assure them, and to create an environment in which their comfort is possible, establish school, synagogue, organizational, and community policies that indicate that their rights and privileges are assured. In addition, establish policies that indicate your intention to be inclusive of people living with AIDS and other people living with "special needs."

5. Learn How Language Has an Impact on the Lives of People Living with AIDS.

Never refer to a person living with AIDS as a "victim" or as a person with a "terminal illness." No one wants to see himself or herself as a victim. A "victim" is someone who has lost control of his or her life, someone who is without power or hope. People living with AIDS have the power and ability to be much more than "victims."

"A person living with a terminal disease" also does not describe a person living with AIDS. People living with terminal diseases are doomed. They have death knocking at their door. They have no hope for a cure, no hope of being able to overcome the obstacles they face.

We use the phrase "people *living* with AIDS" because it emphasizes that they are alive and can continue to live. One of the conditions with which they live is AIDS.

As people of faith, our job is to help restore hope, to provide strength in the face of major challenges. We can't accomplish these things when we talk about "terminal illness." That doesn't mean we should lie or pretend that the illness is not severe. While hope needs to be grounded in each of our realities, each of us is entitled to hope.

Help others understand that language makes a difference. When they talk about victims and terminal illness, they're giving a very wrong and hurtful message.

Psalm 91: 1-2, 4-5, 15-16

O *you who dwell in the shelter of the Most High and abide in the Protection of Shaddai,*

Say of Adonai, my refuge and stonghold, my God in whom I trust, that God will save you. God will cover you with the Holy pinions; you will find refuge under God's wings; God's fidelity is an encircling shield.

You need not fear the terror by night, nor the arrow by day,

the plague that stalks in the darkness, or the scourge that ravages at noon.

When they call on Me, I will answer.

I will be with them when they are in distress;

I will rescue them and make them honored;

I will let them live to a ripe old age, and show them My salvation.

6. Understand What It Means to be Created in the Image of God.

There's a story in the Talmud, *Masechet Derech Eretz* (chapter 4), which relates that once Rabbi Shimon ben Elazar was coming from Migdal Eder, from his teacher's house, and he was riding leisurely on his horse by the seaside. A certain man chanced to meet him, and the man was exceedingly ugly. Rabbi Shimon said to him, "*Raka* (simpleton), how ugly are the children of Abraham our father." The other man replied, "What can I do for you? Speak to the Craftsman Who made me." Rabbi Shimon immediately dismounted from his horse and bowed before the man and said, "I apologize to you, forgive me." He replied to him, "I will not forgive you until you go to the Craftsman Who made me and say, "How ugly is the vessel which You have made."

Rabbi Shimon walked behind him for three miles. When the people in town heard of the arrival of Rabbi Shimon, they came out to meet him and greeted him with the words, "Peace be unto you, rabbi." The other man said to them, "Who are you calling rabbi?" They answered, "The man who is walking behind you." Thereupon he exclaimed, "If this man is a rabbi, may there not be any more like him in Israel!" He told the people the whole story, and they begged him to forgive the rabbi, and he agreed, only on the condition that he never act in this manner again.

The Holy One created all kinds of people. We have to accept, welcome, and love that diversity God created, or else take those issues up with the Creator, not with the person who was created. Diversity is what makes each of us special. Inclusiveness, welcoming, and involvement with the diverse people who share this earth with us make us a holy community. Uniformity is destruction; diversity is our strength and our greatest hope.

It is not up to us to judge people based on the color of their skin, or their gender, or their sexual orientation. If you have a problem with the fact that a person is gay, a woman, or of a different skin color, discuss your problem with the One Who created people to be different, if you're so inclined. But remember that your problem is not with the created but with the Creator.

Gay people in the United States were the "leading edge" of the AIDS epidemic. The government ignored the disease because it was destroying "only" those lives. Unfortunately, religious groups remained silent (or worse, claimed AIDS was "God's will") and did not take on the responsibility to respond in the absence of governmental justice and fairness.

AIDS is not about sexual orientation. AIDS is about disease. The issues of immorality apply to AIDS only when one considers the immorality of people who think they have the right to watch other people suffer and not respond, because those people are somehow "less" or "defective" in some way. *Standing idly by while people are suffering is immoral.*

Claiming that God punishes people through disease is immoral, because (1) it's not true—we dare not say such things about cancer or diabetes or muscular dystrophy; (2) it implies that God is more concerned with the "sin" of homosexuality than with any other sins, which is at best a dubious assumption about God (Imagine if every adulterer or every liar were hit with a plague for these sins!); (3) it deprives people in need of spirituality, of healing, of the very Higher Being they have just as much right to worship and to count on as the religious bigots. No human knows how, if, or when God punishes people at all. It's arrogant to assume that we have such knowledge of the ways in which God works.

AIDS is not about racism. AIDS is about disease. It does not affect minority communities because they are African American or Hispanic. It touches people who transfer body fluids from an infected person into another. AIDS is a symptom of problems faced by the urban poor, such as lack of education, drug abuse, lack of funds and hope—but AIDS is not a result of race.

People involved with people living with AIDS have to deal with their issues of fear of gay people, fear of other races, and fear of people who have been involved with IV drugs. These fears have no basis in reality and can only get in the way. If we are all created in the Divine Image, we share that quality with one another, universally. The image of God is reflected in every human being, and all of God's children deserve and merit God's love and the love of others.

..........*Isaiah 61:7, 8, 9* ....

Because your shame was double,
People cried "Disgrace is their portion."
Assuredly, they shall have a double share in their land,
Joy shall be theirs for all time.
For I, Adonai, love justice and make a covenant with them for all
*   time.*
All who see them shall recognize
That they are a stock Adonai has blessed.

7. Become Familiar with, and Help Others Understand "People with AIDS Bill of Rights"

People with AIDS Bill of Rights

PEOPLE WITH AIDS HAVE THE RIGHT to be treated as living human beings until they die.

PEOPLE WITH AIDS HAVE THE RIGHT not to be discriminated against in housing, courts of law, medical establishments, houses of worship, stores, prisons, or anyplace else.

PEOPLE WITH AIDS HAVE THE RIGHT to maintain a sense of hopefulness, however changing its focus may be.

PEOPLE WITH AIDS HAVE THE RIGHT to be cared for by those who can maintain a sense of hopefulness, however changing its focus may be.

PEOPLE WITH AIDS HAVE THE RIGHT to express feelings and emotions about their approaching deaths in their own ways.

PEOPLE WITH AIDS HAVE THE RIGHT to participate in decisions concerning their care.

PEOPLE WITH AIDS HAVE THE RIGHT to expect continuing medical and nursing attention even if "cure" goals must be changed to "comfort" goals.

PEOPLE WITH AIDS HAVE THE RIGHT not to die alone.

PEOPLE WITH AIDS HAVE THE RIGHT to be free of pain.

PEOPLE WITH AIDS HAVE THE RIGHT to have their questions answered honestly.

PEOPLE WITH AIDS HAVE THE RIGHT not to be deceived.

PEOPLE WITH AIDS HAVE THE RIGHT to have help from, and for, their families in accepting death.

PEOPLE WITH AIDS HAVE THE RIGHT to die in peace and dignity.

PEOPLE WITH AIDS HAVE THE RIGHT to retain their individuality and not be judged for their own decisions, even if those decisions are contrary to others' beliefs.

PEOPLE WITH AIDS HAVE THE RIGHT to discuss and enlarge their religious and spiritual experiences, no matter what these mean to other people.

PEOPLE WITH AIDS HAVE THE RIGHT to expect that the sanctity of the human body will be respected after death.

PEOPLE WITH AIDS HAVE THE RIGHT to be cared for by caring, sensitive, knowledgeable people who attempt to understand their needs.

Source Unknown

8. Understand How to Help the "System"

Many of the programs and services described later in this book benefit people living with AIDS and their caretakers or families. But while many people have the right intentions, they have no idea where to find people living with AIDS whom they can help, or their loved ones. In suburban communities, AIDS is often all but invisible. People who are relatively well and living with AIDS look just like everyone else. Their parents, life companions, siblings, friends and loved ones *are* everyone else, so they are also very difficult to identify. The need for confidentiality is also extreme (see #9), so most of the time people living with AIDS and their caretakers and loved ones are going to have to identify themselves for you to provide services or programs.

When you try to do any of the activities or programs suggested in this book, reach out to numerous people to get the word out to people living with AIDS. Be sure to include people living with AIDS and caretakers on your committee, not only because they will be of tremendous help in finding others with needs for the programs or services you are providing, but also because they *should* be involved in planning a program or service that will serve their needs.

To find the people touched by AIDS in your community, contact AIDS service provider organizations in or close to your community. Describe what you are planning, ask for their reaction and input, and ask for their help in recruitment. Do the same with local health clinics and departments of health. Hospitals generally are not helpful in identifying people living with AIDS, because of the confidentiality of medical records and HIV status, but you may find some help in the chaplain's office or social service staff. Here again, they cannot breach confidentiality rules, but they may be willing to approach people to inform them of your program.

Social service agencies also are bound by confidentiality rules, but they are always searching for programs for their clients to use. Inform their AIDS coordinators or head social workers of what you are planning to offer, and they may suggest that their clients contact you. They will also help you by giving you feedback as to ways to help your program better meet the needs of their clients.

Advertise and submit articles to the local press. Flyers are very helpful, posted in clinics, drug and other stores, hospitals, synagogues and churches, etc.

9. Understand the Need for Confidentiality

People living with AIDS are often subjected to discrimination in health care, housing, food services and insurance. For instance, until the summer of 1993, people who tested HIV positive in New Jersey were denied access to health insurance. Fortunately, that rule has changed in New Jersey, but it hasn't changed in many other states. People living with AIDS face all kinds of both subtle and overt discrimination. Many people live in fear of the reactions of their neighbors, loved ones, or friends to the news of their disease. Whether the fears are based in reality or not, they are real for the person experiencing them and must be respected and honored. (Until you walk in their shoes, you really can't know how they feel.) Not everyone wants to be a symbol; not everyone wants his or her life to be a fight. People who are ill shouldn't have to protest to gain access to basic human rights.

Many states have laws protecting the confidentiality of HIV status and AIDS. Even in states with these guarantees, people living with AIDS have to be on guard that their status will not be revealed to anyone who might ultimately hurt them. Since housing, medical care, or insurance can be denied to a person living with AIDS, they must be allowed to maintain their confidentiality. The implications of a breach in confidentiality may not be readily apparent but could cause unforeseen disasters later on.

This is a challenge, though, because you are trying to set up a program or service to help precisely the people who might want to remain anonymous. In developing your program, plan how you will protect the confidentiality of the people who participate. Plan how you will train your volunteers and participants in guaranteeing the confidentiality of all of your activities and of the people served. If you are setting up a program for delivery of food or phone calls, plan how you will maintain the records of names and addresses and phone numbers in a safe, confidential place, and plan who will have access to those records.

Confidentiality does not apply only to people living with AIDS. Many of the same forms of discrimination are extended to families of people living with AIDS, or their loved ones or caretakers. If you are serving these people in some way, be sure, once again, that their confidentiality is assured. The mother of a person living with AIDS may want to be able to discuss her child's illness without having to worry about the social ostracism that may occur if her identity is revealed in her community.

Establish a policy that your mailing list (if you develop one) will never be for sale or shared with any other organization under any circumstances. The only exception to that rule might be your attachment of mailing labels to another AIDS service provider's mailing, if there is some benefit in the mailing for your participant. Here again, be sure that the envelopes used for mailings also reflect the need for confidentiality. A person living with AIDS in fear of being identified does not need mail coming to his or her home with "AIDS" written on it.

Other AIDS service providers and organizations, as well as mainstream client service providers, will have confidentiality policies. Respect them. They may make your life more difficult in recruiting people to participate in your program, but they are vitally necessary. Encourage the staff people and volunteers of other agencies to recommend your program or service to their clients, and ensure their clients' confidentiality. If a social worker from a hospital tells a person living with AIDS about your program, and that person calls you for more information, there is no breach of confidentiality. Whenever you come upon someone who won't help you find people living with AIDS because of their confidentiality issues, explain that you do not want to breach their confidentiality rules. Rather, you want them to pass along information to their clients, which is something they do all the time.

Section 2: Pikuah Nefesh: Saving Life/Self-protection

According to Jewish law, *pikuah nefesh*, the saving of lives, is more important than anything else. We are commanded to save lives first, even if that means breaking the traditions connected with Shabbat (the day of rest). In the Talmud, *Yoma* 85b, Rabbi Shimon Ben Mansiah declares that we are commanded to sin on Shabbat to save lives so that the people who live as a result of those sins can go on and observe Shabbat later. Saving lives comes first. On the same page, Rabbi Yohanan ben Yosef asserts that the holiness of Shabbat is given into your hands, you are not given into it (to die observing Shabbat). In other words, laws are given for us *to live* by them (*hai bahem*), not die because of them.

From the same principle that saving lives comes first we must extrapolate that while we would prefer to talk with people about sexuality in the context of committed relationships, during the AIDS crisis we have to put saving lives first. Saving lives occurs not only at the last moment when death looms, but also in the long term; AIDS prevention education is saving lives.[2] Just as Rabbi Shimon notes that you save the life first so that people will survive to observe appropriately, we have to save lives first and talk about morality and relationships and all of the other issues of sexuality later on, when we still have people alive to observe.

We are also supposed to protect ourselves from illness. This commandment relates in two ways to the AIDS crisis: the first, as mentioned above, is not to expose ourselves to AIDS, and the second is to understand how to minimize the risk of transmission when you might come into contact

---

[2] It should be noted that another value, *sakanah hamirah d'asurah*, (To prevent onself from danger, one can abrogate commandments) also supports the need for AIDS prevention education. We are clearly commanded to prevent the further spread of AIDS through education, even if that education presupposes that premarital sexual intercourse will be taking place.

with infected body fluids. Understanding the ways in which AIDS is transmitted from one person to another is the the key. *Protecting oneself applies only to real dangers, not to imagined ones.* Therefore, one cannot refuse to sit next to or near a person living with AIDS for fear of "catching it."

Again in the Talmud, *Sanhedrin* 37a says that God created people with one person first (Adam), to "teach you that the loss of any soul among the people of Israel is as though we have lost an entire world. And anyone who saves one life is as though he or she saved an entire world." Further Adam was created singly "so no one could say that his or her father was better than anyone else's." One can mint many coins from the same mold, and each is like another. God, however, made humans from one mold, and yet none is identical to the other. Each and every person has the stamp of the first person, none of them are the same, and yet we are all descendants from the that single source. "Therefore, we are all obligated to say, 'The world was created for me.'"

Saving lives doesn't depend on who one's parents are; it doesn't depend on social status; it doesn't depend on sexual orientation; it doesn't depend on any other criteria. We were all created by God; God created us all alike in our humanity and different in our ways of expressing ourselves and living our lives. We are all the children of the first, single person on earth, precisely so we will realize the value of the things that unify us and love the differences that make each of us special.

Saving a life is like saving an entire world. Is it any wonder that it is more important than anything else?

10. Learn about Risk and Abstinence

While condoms do not work perfectly against the spread of AIDS (some condoms do break, some people use them incorrectly), they are much better than not using any form of barrier against the spread of the disease. Risk should be seen as a continuum from high risk to low risk (see chart below). Behaviors which are high risk should be avoided. We take risks, though, every day, whether driving our cars or crossing the street. We judge some risks to be worth taking; some risks are too scary. So, too, with "safe sex." The risk involved in unprotected (without a condom) anal or vaginal intercourse should be considered too great for anyone to take. The risk involved in protected (using a condom) anal or vaginal intercourse is significantly decreased.

We also should be honest with people about sexual behaviors that do not involve any risk of transmission of AIDS whatsoever. You can't get AIDS from mutual masturbation, hugging, petting, massage or any other sexual activity which does not involve the exchange of bodily fluids (though if there are open wounds on the skin, and one of the partners is actively bleeding, there is some risk). Some people may not feel comfortable telling teenagers that they can masturbate together, but their reasons have nothing to do with AIDS.

High Risk
Unprotected anal intercourse (without a condom)
Unprotected vaginal intercourse (without a condom)
Sharing any sexual "toys" such as dildos or vibrators.

Considered less risky

Anal intercourse using a condom (and withdrawal prior to ejaculation)

Vaginal intercourse using a condom (and withdrawal prior to ejaculation)

Oral/penile sex (Condoms are recommended. The risk is from semen or preseminal fluid entering the bloodstream through small sores or cuts in the mouth.)

Oral/vaginal intercourse (A dental dam is recommended to prevent vaginal secretions from entering the bloodstream through small sores or cuts in the mouth.)

Oral/rectal intercourse (A dental dam is recommended.)

No Risk

Massage/Hugging

Masturbation (alone or with partners)

Kissing

Using sexual toys personally (without sharing)

Any other activities that don't let blood, semen, or vaginal secretions into another person's body

Abstinence

Preaching abstinence doesn't work and is, therefore, a highly risky behavior. It's risky because it makes the person preaching it look irrelevant, uninformed, and unreliable. While I have consistently told teenagers that they do not have my or their parents' permission to engage in sexual activity, I want them to have the information necessary to survive their own errors. I don't think we will ever convince teenagers not to have sexual relations (just as I don't think we'll be able to convince unmarried adults not to have sex). We know that over 80% of all teenagers have had sexual relations by the age of 19; over 50% by the age of 15.

We have to get real in the face of this crisis. Getting real means being willing to talk to people about things that make us personally uncomfortable, but may save lives. Preaching abstinence *exclusively* is not real. Anyone who thinks he or she can convince someone not to engage in any form of sexual relations "because I said so" is only fooling him or herself and endangering the life of the person receiving only that message, because that person will not have the information necessary to avoid the risk of infection.

Preaching abstinence exclusively is a smoke screen for real AIDS prevention education. It shows a lack of comfort in talking openly and honestly about issues related to sexuality and attempts to hide that insecurity. Abstinence is being used to teach sexual morality with AIDS as a punishment for sexual activity. In a time of crisis, when lives are at stake, we are clearly instructed by the rabbis to save lives first, teach morality later.

Abstinence does have a place in overall AIDS prevention education. It should always be a part of what is taught; we do have an obligation to encourage people to abstain from sexual intercourse outside of meaningful relationships. But teaching abstinence is only one component in the education that must take place.

11. Develop an AIDS Prevention Educational Program for Teenagers ....

If you are a member or leader of a congregation that hasn't done this yet, it's essential. It's important for teenagers to get the message from all possible directions, including the rabbi or other clergy, parents and teachers. It's important for you as a concerned leader or member, to know that the message is appropriate, honest and reliable. It's important for the message to include the specific religious values that make AIDS a religious issue.

The following is an outline for a four-hour workshop for teenagers and their parents. You should feel free to adapt this outline to your own school and setting. I recommend bringing a person living with AIDS to participate in your workshop. The person should be willing and able to talk about anything related to the experience of living with AIDS and how AIDS is spread. Be sure he or she is open to answer very personal questions. You can get a person living with AIDS to serve as your speaker by contacting AIDS service provider organizations in your local area. Most have speakers' bureaus or will be willing to make a few contacts for you. If possible, it's good to have a speaker of the same religious background as your target audience, and relatively close to their age. (In speaking to teenagers, it's most effective to find a person living with AIDS who got it in high school. Unfortunately, this population of people living with AIDS is growing rapidly.)

It is advantageous to have parents and teenagers participate simultaneously in these workshops. This (1) stimulates informed conversation at home; (2) provides parents with accurate and reliable AIDS prevention information that may be necessary for their own sexual activity; (3) allows parents to know precisely what was said to their children, so they can respond to it and add their own input. While parents may object to their children's participation in this kind of workshop without their presence, they will often attend with their children.

You may find program ideas and information that will be useful for your workshops elsewhere in this book.

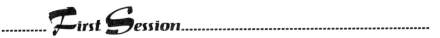

I. Introduction: AIDS 101 for Parents and Teens (30 minutes)

A. Define AIDS.

B. Define HIV.

C. Discuss means of transmission of HIV from one person to another. (Exchange of bodily fluids, particularly semen, vaginal secretions, blood or breast milk, with another person. Be specific on how these fluids can go from one person to another. Define sexual intercourse as the insertion of a penis into any other person's bodily orifices, such as a mouth, vagina or anus. This is not the time to be shy about sexual relations! Your specific instructions now can save lives later.)

D. Discuss ways AIDS is not spread from one person to another. (Low concentrations of HIV in other body fluids: you would need to drink 40 buckets of tears to expose a person to a significant concentration of HIV. AIDS can't be spread by sweat, saliva, unclean public toilet seats, etc.)

E. Discuss how AIDS is spread through intravenous drug use.

    1. Do not share needles with anyone for any reason.

    2. Note that IV drugs themselves are not the issue in the transmission of AIDS. It's not the drugs that spread AIDS, it's sharing needles. (Some people think that sharing needles for steroid use is okay. We have to dispel that myth! Also note that some people use hypodermic needles for the wrong purposes, like piercing ears. Here again, ear piercing is not the problem or the risk; passing the needle from person to person is.)

F. Emphasize that you are not giving anyone *permission* to engage in sexual activity or intravenous drug use. That permission is not your job. You are there to tell people how they can protect themselves from a disease that is preventable with the proper education.

G. Emphasize that there is no risk of transmission of the AIDS virus when there is no sexual contact. Say it a few times so the parents hear the abstinence message; they need to hear it, though the teenagers will not.

H. Note that sexual intercourse, the behavior that involves a high level of risk for exposure for AIDS, requires the use of condoms. If people want to engage in other forms of sexual contact, that do not involve the insertion of any body parts into another person, those behaviors pose no risk for transmission of the AIDS virus. (It's not enough to say that people should abstain. They won't. Better you should provide other alternatives as well.)

II. Living with AIDS (30 minutes)

A. Introduce the person living with AIDS and allow him or her to tell his or her personal story. If you do not have a person living with AIDS available, use a videotape and discuss it afterward.[3]

B. Discuss with the person living with AIDS the challenges for people living with AIDS in your local community. Be sure to ask what people living with AIDS need, want, or could use.

III. Smaller discussion groups (30 minutes)

A. Teenagers meet with the person living with AIDS to ask any questions they have about his or her life, living with AIDS, and AIDS prevention. It is preferable for the teenagers to meet with this person without any other adults present, if possible. When parents, teachers, or clergy members sit in on the discussion, the teenagers are less likely to ask the kinds of questions they would in the absence of other authority figures. The person with AIDS is there to make sure that

---

[3] You can get very good videos from your local department of health, AIDS service providers, national or regional offices of your religious denomination. I have not provided a listing of videos because there is such a wide variety of videos available, and they constantly change. New ones become available on a daily basis. In looking for a good video, seek one which reiterates most of the AIDS 101 information you have already presented and which introduces the audience to the personal experiences of people living with AIDS. Teachers should always view videos prior to showing them to their classes.

the teenagers get the message. Few educators have such an ability to transmit the lifesaving knowledge, and few can speak with such conviction or so knowledgeably. Trust that the session will be on target and appropriate, even in discussing sex and drugs. The last thing a person living with AIDS is going to do is encourage behavior that could put another person in the same situation.

B. Parents meet with teaching staff and presenter(s) to discuss parenting issues related to AIDS. While many parents may claim to have the ability to discuss AIDS with their children, many may not have the skills necessary. Discuss the issues that cause the most anxiety for parents. In particular, emphasize that you are not giving children *permission* to do *anything.* Discussion of their sexuality is not *permission* for teenagers to engage in sexual activity. The parents and the teachers are just attempting to influence the behavior of teenagers, most of whom, despite their parents' wishes and the advice of every adult they know, engage in sexual activity. Role-playing is sometimes helpful, focusing on what both the parent and teenager got out of the workshop.

The other major emphasis of this session is to discuss access to condoms. Now that parents understand that their children's lives depend on the use of condoms, they also have to understand that they have to assist their children in gaining access to this protection.

Many parents have told me that they gave their *son* a condom, when the son was 15 or so. I point out to the parents that since they gave their son this one condom, two years ago, it has been in a wallet, which the son has been sitting on for hours each day. The condom is probably no good anymore because of that kind of abuse. One also has to wonder whether access to one condom is ever enough. What if it breaks or is torn by nervous fingers? Do parents really imagine their children will get into a position where they need a condom and will stop the sexual activity the minute they realize that the condom is no good? Not too likely. People don't generally think that well in the heat of passion.

The hardest thing for a teenager to do, particularly a young woman, is to go to a drug store and buy condoms. Male teenagers can do it with less difficulty, because our society enables them to put on a "macho" act

45

But young women are often too embarrassed even to purchase personal feminine hygiene products. Condoms are just out of the question. If we want teenagers to take the message seriously, we have to enable them to gain access to the condoms at the same time we remind them that we would prefer that they not get into situations in which they need them.

I am suggesting a very mixed message. But there are few good alternatives for parents. They can ignore the issue, and risk their child's acquiring the AIDS virus because of a lack of information, or they can make condoms available. By available I mean a discreet bowl somewhere at home containing an uncounted number of condoms, and no questions asked when the bowl looks like it needs refilling. (Would a parent prefer the use of the condoms in the bowl? If they're not safe, free of any feedback from a parent, and easily accessible, a teenager won't use them. Think of it as analogous to the deal parents are supposed to make with their teenagers about drunk driving. If the teen gets drunk and shouldn't drive, and contacts the parents, they are supposed to pick the teenager up, no questions asked. In this way, the teenager arrives home alive, and the parent can rest assured that at least the teenager is not going to drive when his or her judgment is impaired.)

IV. Wrap-up for first session (30 minutes)

Bring both groups together and have a general discussion about what people learned and what they still need to know. Answer remaining questions. Assign homework: Ask the teenagers to bring in any articles about AIDS from any news media in the period of time between the first and second sessions. Wish the parents good luck.

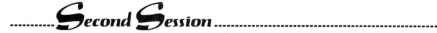
Second Session

V. Review homework (45 minutes)

I like to do a values clarification game for the review if the group is over 20 people. This game is an adaptation of one that I learned from Dr. Jeffrey Spector, who did it at a workshop for the Bureau of Jewish Education in MetroWest, NJ. The game is called "Four Questions." Prepare in advance index cards, one per person, as follows (based on 20 people—for more or less, adjust the number of cards accordingly): Place a small, discreet "a" on 2 cards; an "s" on 2 cards; a "d" on 3 cards; a "c" on 2 cards. Give each person a card, and tell them to ignore any letters that might be on them. Ask the people to get into groups of 4, and tell them all they have to do is write down the names of the people they meet with in each group. Once the participants are in their groups and have written down the names of the other people in their group, ask them to summarize the newspaper or magazine article on AIDS that they brought in for their group. Each group has about 2 minutes, after which they get into completely new groups of 4. Again, they write down only the names of the people in their new group on their cards. Ask any question for discussion, such as: Should more money go for AIDS research or for prevention education if you only have limited funds? What would you do if your friend told you he or she was having unprotected sexual intercourse? How would your parents react to the news that a classmate of yours has AIDS? What would you do if a relative told you he or she has AIDS? (The questions really don't matter for the purposes of the game, though good thought-provoking and discussion-provoking questions would be the best use of the time.) Repeat this procedure for four rounds, so all participants have a total of 12 names on their cards (4 rounds times the three other people in each group).

After the fourth round, ask the people with "a" written on their cards to stand. These people have full-blown AIDS. They have all been in contact with the people on their cards. Ask them to read the names of the people on their cards, and have the people whose names are read stand. This should get almost everyone standing. Now ask the people who have a "c" on their cards to sit down. They used a condom. People with a "d" on their cards can also sit down; they didn't do anything (abstained). People with an "s" engaged in safe sex and can also sit. The people remaining standing have been exposed.

Ask all of the people with the letters how they felt. Ask the people who were still standing at the end how they felt about it. Discuss the reactions. Note that there were only 2 people with "a" cards at the beginning. Also note that all of the people who were still standing also came into contact with other people who may not have been read off by the people with the "a" cards, but their exposure was just as real. Discuss all of the implications of the game for the group.

Ask whether there are any other questions about how AIDS is transmitted from person to person.

VI. Jewish Values (30 minutes)

While all phases of the workshop focus on Jewish values, they may not have been emphasized specifically. Refer to the five sections of this book: *Talmud Torah* (learning), *Pikuah Nefesh* (saving lives), *Bikkur Holim* (visiting the sick), *Shituf B'tsaar* (alleviating another's pain) and *Tikkun Olam* (making the world a better place), and discuss all of these values with the teenagers. Break into small groups; assign each group one of these values. They have ten minutes to come up with an example of this value being put into action with regard to someone living with AIDS, and to develop their idea into a short role-play. Have each of the groups present their skit for the others, and ask the audience to figure out which Jewish value is being portrayed. Review all of the plays for authenticity of the situation depicted and discuss the thought processes that went into the skits.

VII. Helping People Living with AIDS (30 minutes)

I believe the best way to reinforce the message on a regular basis is to provide the participants with an ongoing social action project they can continue throughout the school year. The easiest one to develop is a drive for personal, household, or over-the-counter medical products for people living with AIDS (See Ways 30-33).

This social action project should be exclusively a project of the teenagers. If they can be the leadership for a congregation-wide program, that's also great. Be sure to review the reasons these items are necessary, and the value of helping others who are in need. Set a date for the first collection to be completed. Have the participants develop a leadership plan for the collection (i.e., who is in charge of contacting an AIDS service provider organization to let them know you will have supplies; who will contact local press and the congregational newsletter; who will make announcements at services and congregational events; who should receive phone calls about the project).

VIII. Review everything

Remind the participants that if they have any further questions about AIDS or how they can help, all they have to do is call you. Thank them for their cooperation and involvement.

12. Help Combat the Myths, Misinformation, and Prejudice Associated with AIDS

Wear a red ribbon.

One of the most important things you can do in getting started to help people living with AIDS is to wear a red ribbon at all times. Red ribbons indicate that you are "AIDS friendly." You care about helping people living with AIDS; you are informed about AIDS; you are willing and able to do something to help other people; you have contributed to an AIDS service provider organization; you will not tolerate AIDS phobia or bigotry.

Wearing a red ribbon puts a lot of messages in the eyes of people who see you. People living with AIDS or loving a person living with AIDS, or who have lost a loved one to AIDS, will see you and know that you are with them. Some will approach you and ask questions about AIDS or how to access help. Some will tell you of their commitment or involvement. Some will invite you to an event or a meeting. A world of possibilities opens when you wear your ribbon.

When you're asked what the ribbon means (and you *will* be asked), say, "It means I care about people living with AIDS." Observe the reaction, and follow up the reaction with conversation.

By wearing a red ribbon you become a goodwill ambassador, educating people about AIDS, signifying that AIDS affects all of us, and providing visibility for concern about the disease where you live. Just by wearing the ribbon you will be helping to eliminate AIDS bigotry and AIDS phobia. At the same time that you will be invited, informally, to provide information to people in need of assistance. They may not say anything to you; just know that they're out there looking, and their hearts are warmed by your ribbon.

13. Develop an AIDS Resource Center

Many congregations have libraries, including all kinds of religious books. Consider adding books, pamphlets, magazines and videos on topics related to AIDS to your collection. Include AIDS prevention, living with a person living with AIDS, spirituality and AIDS, and survival techniques. Include other resources that touch on the epidemic as well, such as guides for visiting the sick or visiting the homes of people who are bereaved. Emphasize those items that directly relate to your religious denomination, but have general information available as well.

This resource center will be of tremendous help to people living with AIDS in your community, as well as to their families and loved ones and people of faith who may not have someone living with AIDS in their immediate families or social circles, but who care deeply and want to help.

Consider asking a person living with AIDS or a loved one to develop and run this resource center. This kind of project could be very helpful in keeping a person living with AIDS challenged on a very part-time volunteer basis or could be a positive way to channel grief for people who have lost a loved one.

Many of these resources are available free of charge, or for a very limited amount of money. Funding for this kind of resource center could come from all sorts of sources, such as a special fund-raising event, a few donors who want to create a living memorial for a loved one, or central funding sources (such as Jewish Federation or United Way). A community-wide AIDS Resource Center, housed in one congregation but involving other local congregations, could also seek funding from all of the other local congregations.

Section 3: Bikkur Holim: Visiting the Sick

Rabbi Aha, son of Rabbi Haninah, once said, "Anyone who visits a sick person carries away with him/her one sixtieth of the illness" (*Nedarim* 39b). Rabbi Akiva said that anyone who does not visit the sick "is like someone who sheds blood." Rabbi Akiva makes it very clear that when we can be helpful, we must be, or it's as if we were intentionally harming someone. Visiting the sick is considered to be one of the biggest mitzvot (commandments/good deeds) you can do.

Visiting the sick helps people who are ill feel less alone or frightened. It alleviates some of the symptoms of their disease, eases their pain, helps them focus on other things than their own suffering, or allows them to unburden themselves of some of the hurt. Visiting the sick can be an uplifting experience both for the person who is ill and for the person who is visiting. What could be more meaningful than knowing you have done something to help a person who is suffering?

If you don't personally know someone living with AIDS who would like to be visited, volunteer for a AIDS service provider organization. You'll meet plenty of people who will benefit from your assistance and who will also need to be visited at one time or another. If you would like to visit people immediately, there are organizations (like Buddies[4] groups) that train volunteers for journeying with a person living with AIDS, and still other AIDS service organizations in your community that might know of someone who could use a visit. Because of confidentiality rules, hospitals are not allowed to disclose who is living with AIDS

---

[4]Buddies groups are available in many communities, and train volunteers extensively in how to work with a "buddy" living with AIDS. They pair people living with AIDS with volunteers who help their buddies in any way necessary, whether it's with shopping, companionship, laundry, or whatever the people living with AIDS need.

and in the hospital, but if you contact the chaplain's office, and let them know you are available for visiting in the hospital and would like to help people living with AIDS in particular, they will often ask the patients whether a visit from a volunteer will be welcomed.

If you are intimidated by the idea of visiting someone who is in a hospital, nursing home, or homebound or bedbound, I have included in this section ways in which you will also be able to "visit" the sick without getting into situations that are still too hard for you.

The important thing is to offer and provide help for someone who is ill, to alleviate some of their illness, to remove at least one sixtieth of the illness by your presence and/or involvement.

Isaiah 58:8-9, 11

*Then shall your light burst through like the dawn
And your healing spring up quickly;
Your Vindicator shall march before you;
The Presence of Adonai shall be your rear guard,
Then, when you call, Adonai will answer;
When you cry, God will say, "Here I am."
Then shall your light shine in darkness,
And your gloom shall be like noonday. Adonai will guide you always,
And will give strength to your bones.*

14. When You Visit

Call first

I f you're visiting a person at home, it's always preferable to call first and allow the person who is ill to determine when would be the best time for your visit. Even when a person is in a hospital, if he or she has a phone, call first. People living with AIDS often do not know from day to day what they will feel like, and in the hospital they have even less ability to control their schedule. You don't want to visit precisely when he or she is due to go for physical therapy or to a special room for a test of some kind. Always check during your phone call whether there is anything the person needs that you can pick up on your way over.

Prepare for your visit

Because of the wide variety of opportunistic infections that people living with AIDS confront, find out what, specifically, he or she is facing, and read up on the symptoms so you know what to expect. A person living with PCP or other respiratory problems may be coughing or spitting up phlegm, may have an oxygen tube, etc. Talking may be a challenge for him or her (hearing may not be a problem, and may just be soothing). A person living with major skin fungi or infections may be itchy, unable to sit still very long, agitated, uncomfortable. Bringing books for people who are going blind from CMV may be an embarrassing experience, while a book on tape might be deeply appreciated. A little preparation will help you be a good visitor.

Wash your hands

Do you know where your hands have been? What you've touched today could be filled with all kinds of germs you don't need to bring with you to visit a person whose immune system is compromised. Leave the germs in the sink!

Know what you're there for

You are visiting to help raise someone's spirits, to unburden this person of some of the pain, to offer a helping hand. You are not the medical professional. If a nurse tells you he or she needs to see the patient alone, go. If you don't like a specific form of treatment, or if you object to a therapy, it's not your place to argue with the doctors or nurses. Medical decisions are made by medical professionals in consultation with their patients. You have no place in that equation. If the patient has a problem and includes you, by asking for your help, then and only then have you a right to act as an advocate for the patient. You can discuss what the doctors and nurses are doing if your friend in the bed wants to discuss it. Otherwise, it's none of your business. Your are not there to question the therapies the doctor has chosen or to shake your friend's confidence in the doctor. That relationship is one in which your friend has been involved for a while. His or her confidence and trust in his or her medical professional is extremely important.

Sometimes knowing your place is hard. When my friend Michael was in the hospital for his last six months, he was in what the hospital called "respiratory isolation." People entering his room were supposed to wear masks, and Michael was not permitted to leave his room at all, ever. As winter turned to spring I asked Michael whether he wouldn't just like to go and sit outside for a few minutes. He told me he wasn't allowed to leave his room, and he didn't want to argue with the medical and nursing staff. Though his isolation was exclusively for the convenience of the institution and was a part of AIDS phobia, I had to accept Michael's wishes. If he had said yes, I also would have respected his wishes and fought with the staff for him to be allowed to cover his face and go outside. It was Michael's life, and Michael's decision. Now that he's no longer suffering, it's my job to go back to the hospital staff and see that future patients living with AIDS are not treated in the same way.

On the other hand, when I saw that my friend Richard's loss of weight was both rapid and dramatic, I insisted he discuss it with his doctor, and I suggested that they talk about dietary supplements and Marinol (the marijuana derivative that can help improve the appetite). Once the doctor agreed it would help, I picked up the prescription for Richard. While

I thought Richard's doctor was less than competent, Richard trusted him, so I worked with Richard in pointing the doctor in the right direction.

Help or get out of the way

There are times when you visit that you are called on to do all kinds of work you never expected to do. For instance, you might be asked to help feed people who are too weak, or whose coordination is impaired by either neuropathies or drugs; you might be asked to rub a back or a leg, or to help someone walk to the bathroom, hallway, etc. Sometimes the most appreciated gesture is in the practical assistance you can give, the personal touch, the run to the corner for an iced tea or ice cream sandwich. Be there for whatever is needed. For me, so far, the most extreme and strange assistance I had to offer was to help a nurse with a urinary catheter. She needed another set of hands, my friend was very uncomfortable, and the sooner the catheter was inserted, the better. My friend in the bed was more concerned with getting the catheter going than with his privacy. (He also thought having me assist was funny. The shared experience did bring us closer.)

Self-protection

If you are called upon to offer technical assistance, remember you will need to put on gloves if there is even the remotest chance of coming into contact with any bodily fluids. If you are changing a dressing on a wound, emptying a urinal, getting rid of used tissues, or helping in any other way in which you might come into contact with bodily fluids, put the gloves on. (This is actually a medical overreaction, but what could it hurt?)

If you are visiting a person with active tuberculosis or other respiratory ailments and the nurses say put on a mask, put it on and keep it on. People with healthy immune systems generally will not catch anything from a person living with AIDS, but some strains of tuberculosis seem to be potential risks.

You do not need gloves for feeding a person, for rubbing his/her skin (unless it's bleeding, in which case, why are you rubbing?), offering drinks, cleaning used dishes or cups, laundry, etc.

Don't make things worse

Never, never visit a person living with AIDS if you are ill or were recently exposed to a cold, chicken pox, or any other disease.

If you have a cold, you are carrying germs that could literally kill a person living with AIDS. Stay home. Get well. If you don't listen to this sage advice, be sure to put on a mask, wash your hands thoroughly prior to entering the environment of a person living with AIDS, and don't cough or sneeze or leave your tissues anywhere. Remember that the immune system is what keeps people well. People living with AIDS don't have the ability to fight off the diseases other people can fight off. They also lose their immunity to childhood diseases, like chicken pox, which becomes shingles in people living with AIDS. If you're around children, be careful about what you may be carrying with you to people living with AIDS. When you call, if you suspect a problem, ask them to ask their doctor if it's okay for you to visit.

Know when to leave

The rabbis (in *Nedarim* 51a) warn us that the visitor must be careful not to be a burden to the person who is ill. Be careful not to stay too long. If the person seems tired, ask whether you should stay until he or she falls asleep. (I have found that many people who are taking heavy-duty drugs that make them drowsy prefer not to be alone when they fall asleep.) By offering to stay, you (1) acknowledge that it's okay for the person to fall asleep, and (2) get some feedback on whether you should stay. Always respect what the person tells you to do.

Don't stick around, unless you are asked to, for medical procedures or for bodily functions. If your visit is over, go. If it's not, go get something the person in the bed needs, and come back later.

When are you coming back?

When my friend Mel was in the hospital for his last time, I went to visit. At the end of the visit he asked when I was coming back. He did that every time I came to see him, until his last night, when he knew, as I did, that I would not be back. (Mel died around 4:30 A.M. I was the last person to be with him, when I left at 11:00 P.M. I believe people die when they are ready. Mel died when there was no one around so no one would run for a nurse and maybe bring him back and prolong the suffering.)

You don't have to be there every day. You don't have to be there even every week. You get to set the pace of your involvement. This is important for you. Don't take on more than you can handle, or you won't be helpful for very long. So answer the question in a way that fits for you.

---------- *Psalm 121:8* --

Adonai will bless your going out and your coming in now and forever.

15. Bring Food to Someone Who Is Homebound or in the Hospital

You don't even have to visit to make a nice bowl of chicken soup, or meat loaf, or some chopped liver. Nothing is worse than depending on the kitchen of a hospital for good, tasty, healthy food (ironic, no?). Make a few extra matzah balls, a little extra soup, and bring them to a person living with AIDS. A visit may remove a sixtieth of the illness, but a bowl of chicken soup with matzah balls is good for at least twice that!

When my friend Richard was released from the hospital there was no way he could prepare food for himself, except what he could nuke in the microwave. He was just too weak to cook. I called Rabbi Glazer, who had referred Richard to me in the first place, and asked if he could find a nice Jewish mother in his congregation who would be willing to make a meal for Richard every few days. Rabbi Glazer immediately said, "Sure." Every Shabbat, while Richard was still able to eat, a different person brought a meal to his home. Most meals lasted him days. Richard loved the food, but almost more importantly, he loved this kindness of strangers. Rabbi Glazer and the Fair Lawn Jewish Center showed Richard that there were people all around him who cared and who were willing to put in a little effort to help keep him alive. It made a huge difference for him.

16. Bring Something to Do

What could be more boring than sitting around all day, feeling crummy, and watching TV? There are only so many talk shows and soaps you can watch before your brain goes dead. So help people who are sick fight the boredom by bringing them things to do with their hands. (This won't work for everyone, but it will work for some.) Try jigsaw puzzles, Rubik's cubes or similar games, crossword puzzles, anything you see in the adult section of a toy store that could be useful. If the person you're visiting has neuropathy in his or her hands, get some Silly Putty, clay, Play Doh, whatever—perhaps one of the "tension releasing" things that you squeeze in your hands—anything to get their hand muscles moving so they don't completely atrophy.

For people who have relatively good eye-hand coordination, have someone teach them how to knit, crochet, do origami, or create something with their hands. The point is to keep their minds working, allow for creativity, lessen the boredom, create opportunities that give people a chance to contribute despite their illness. Find an AIDS service provider organization that needs envelopes stuffed, pick them up, drop them off. Few people want to lose their usefulness. But beware: Even when they're feeling crummy, they can still roll Silly Putty into a ball to throw at the visitor who brought it!

Books and magazines are good, too, but many people who are taking heavy-duty drugs, or battling opportunistic infections like CMV that destroy the eyesight, can't use books. Books on tape are great for people whose eyes are failing. They are relatively inexpensive and are reusable. Many libraries now stock books on tape as well. Find out what kind of literature your friend likes, and help him or her access it on tape. Listen to the tape yourself so you can discuss the story.

17. Make Phone Calls to People Living with AIDS

Don't assume every homebound person with AIDS has someone who is looking in on him or her every day. Even if one does have a visitor every day, it can be very lonely—when the visitor is gone, when the TV programs are boring or heavy, or when the mail is filled with particularly depressing bills.

A simple phone call can make a person's day. It can be the responsibility of one person or a team of people. Call. Check in. Take care of any needs that arise during the conversation. But most important, listen and share.

To get the phone number of a person living with AIDS who would appreciate a daily phone call, contact your local AIDS service provider organization. They may not have a list readily available, though (because no one else has offered to do the calls). Offer your help in developing the list.

18. Develop a Phone Team for Daily Conversations with People Living with AIDS

Systems have been developed for elderly people to receive a phone call every day to make sure they're okay. The same kind of system could be developed for people living at home with AIDS. This could be a school or congregation-wide social action project. Gather a corps of people interested in being phone supporters. Contact AIDS service provider organizations to let them know that you're developing this kind of a program and that you have volunteers willing to make daily phone contact with their clients living with AIDS. When you find an agency that is interested in working with you, they will train your volunteers, poll their clients, and give you the numbers of people who would like the calls. (If the agency says they can't provide you with phone numbers because of confidentiality, just tell them that they have to contact the clients first, ask if they want this service, and get their permission for release of their phone number.) Agencies interested in seeing this program happen will do it.

To get other phone numbers, set up a table at a function for people living with AIDS, their loved ones, and their caregivers, or at a local AIDS clinic, and the names and numbers will come to you.

The phone squad can work in various ways. Each person in the squad may take one number and call daily, or seven people could each call the list of numbers once a week on an assigned day, or any combination thereof. The squad's purpose is simply to talk to people living with AIDS who are homebound. However, callers should also be ready to respond to other needs people have as they make contact (which could mean referrals for other services or programs).

19. Visit and Provide Breaks for Primary Caretakers

It's so hard to watch a loved one suffer. It's hard, terrible and terrifying work to watch the body of a loved one deteriorate to the point of death. It's heartbreaking to watch hopes and dreams disappear, and to be virtually powerless against the relentless attack on a loved one's life.

Despite the impossibility of the task, mothers and fathers, brothers and sisters, lovers and friends have taken on these kinds of responsibilities, sacrificing years of their own lives to ease the pain and devastation for their loved ones. Many primary caretakers have other responsibilities as well, like other family members, jobs, their own health and well-being.

Sometimes the best way to help the person who is ill is to help the caretaker with the caretaker's needs. When a mother is focusing all of her time and efforts on her dying son, you can assist with meals for the other family members, baby-sitting, household chores, shopping and errands. Visit the caretaker and offer whatever assistance you can give. It doesn't have to be a big deal. Walking someone's dog so he or she doesn't have to rush home to care for the family pet can make a huge difference in reducing tension and anxiety.

Primary caretakers tend to ignore their own needs. Look at the frazzled caretaker and see what personal needs he or she is leaving unmet. Then help the caretaker to see what needs to be done and help implement a plan. A caretaker who is frazzled will inevitably burn out from the self-neglect and will give out all kinds of inadvertent, unconscious messages to the person in the bed. Your care and attention for the caretaker will have a positive, though indirect, impact on the person living with AIDS.

I always marveled at the way Florence was with Steve his last year. She was always there when he was at home (his apartment) or when he was in the hospital. She was always cheerful and positive, even when Steve was gloomy. One day, when Steve was undergoing yet another test that would predict his death, I sat with Florence, chatted with her, and held her as she cried. I was glad I was there, even though I didn't see Steve at all that day.

20. Cards, Flowers, Plants, Things to Brighten a Bleak Room

Flowers are always welcome. Silk flowers don't wilt and can send a very positive message about human life not fading away. Plants, especially plants that bloom, also send a message of renewal and hope as they brighten a room. Mylar balloons can make for something to do. Cards can brighten a room, lifting the spirits of a person living with AIDS.

Many people are afraid to send get-well cards to a person with a "terminal" illness. As Yogi Berra said, "It ain't over 'till it's over." Good wishes are appropriate at all times. Word your card with care if recovery does not seem possible; renewed strength, healing, peace, are all words that can be hopeful and helpful in the face of imminent death. Just don't give up on the helpfulness of any of these messages, even in the last days of a person's life. The transition to the next world is a scary one for all of us. Wishes for peace, inner healing, and faith can help ease the transition, plus the messages may be helpful for the caretakers and survivors who are sharing the same time and space.

Cards and decorations for the living spaces of people living with AIDS can be a terrific class or group project and can be delivered to hospitals or through AIDS service provider organizations.

21. Make Warm, Fuzzy Items for People Living with AIDS.

Those people who are creative can make all kinds of things that are useful and meaningful for people living with AIDS. One nursing home in New Jersey is producing lap blankets and afghans for people who are hospitalized. It's a great project, giving the elderly in the nursing homes an opportunity to help others in need. Students in the art program of one school made soft sculptures (teddy bears) as a project; all of their bears were donated to people living with AIDS. (Not just children; sometimes, when you're stuck in a bed all day, it's good for even an adult to squeeze a teddy bear.) When one considers the impersonal nature of life in a hospital, a handmade lap blanket, afghan, or stuffed animal can add a lovely note of warmth. When the person goes home this lap blanket, afghan, or stuffed animal will be one of the precious things the person will actually take home from the hospital.

Consider the kinds of hobbies you have and the possibility of using your hobby to benefit a person living with AIDS. Your only limitation is your imagination.

Any hospital will be willing to distribute this kind of gift to a person living with AIDS. If you attach a card with a phone number for the person receiving the gift to call if he or she needs anything, it could start you on other projects included in this book. The card could also have a nice message about healing and peace, and an address to send a thank-you card to.

22. Hold Drives to Collect Books, Tapes and Games

Hold a book, audiotape, books-on-tape, and/or games drive to collect these items and donate them to an AIDS service provider organization, hospital, or nursing home with a population of people living with AIDS. Medical establishments are most concerned with the physical well-being of the patients and do not necessarily pay much attention to their spirits and their interests, particularly long-term chronic care facilities. It is in precisely these facilities, though, that residents need diversions from their boredom.

Books of interest are often scarce, and paperbacks fall apart. After you finish the novels you read, donate them where they could be put to use rather than sitting on a bookshelf for a few years. (I almost never reread a suspense thriller. Once you know how it ends, what's the point of keeping it?)

If you hold a book drive, be specific as to the kinds of books you want. I doubt that economics textbooks from the 1960s will be useful. Tastes do vary, but emphasize readable, interesting books in good condition.

I have an extensive collection of audiotapes that I never listen to, since I never turn off the CD player. The tapes are still good, and I should have donated them long ago. Since I haven't turned on my tape deck for more than two years, I'm probably not going to. Tape players are much more portable than CD players, and more easily accessible to people in hospitals.

One local transitional housing program for homeless people living with AIDS needed board games for residents to play. Great idea. But of course, their state funding did not include any activities funds. One church donated new sets of Monopoly, Scrabble, Risk, cards, etc. If you're no longer playing your board games, and they're still in good shape and have all their pieces, consider giving them to a place where they will actually get some use.

Hold a drive for all of these items, and give them to a place where they might be used and appreciated.

23. Provide Transportation

If you want to help fulfill the mitzvah of visiting the sick, but you just can't handle the actual visit, help someone who can. Provide transportation for someone to visit a loved one living with AIDS in the hospital or nursing home. Many people don't drive or don't own cars. In northern New Jersey, the largest nursing home for people living with AIDS was built in the middle of nowhere, with no way to get there by public transportation. (That's not really true. There is a bus to and from New York City. So people who live in Newark can take the bus into the city about one-half hour, change buses, and ride for another hour and a half to the nursing home. Those people who have two hours for a forty-minute car trip might actually do this. I wouldn't.) Many of the residents have come to this home because it is the last and only place that can deal with their medical needs, and they have no alternatives. Their relatives are often in the inner cities in New Jersey.

Developing transportation for these people could be extremely helpful. In your own community, call the local hospitals and ask the social worker or chaplain's office if there is a need for this kind of assistance. Let them know you're volunteering. If they don't express an immediate need, they will, once they know you're available. Contact any nursing homes with people living with AIDS and ask whether they need this kind of assistance.

In addition, contact your local AIDS service provider organizations and let them know you are available to drive people who want to visit the sick. There are a lot of volunteers out there who would love to have the opportunity to visit the sick but have no way to get there. Team up with them.

24. Develop a Bikkur Holim (Visiting the Sick) Committee

Developing a *Bikkur Holim* Committee to share the communal responsibility of visiting the sick could help all members of your congregation who are ill, including people who are living with AIDS. The committee would be notified by members of the family or friends of a person who is ill of any special needs the person has (visits, food, transportation, etc.). The committee would contact the clergy and assign a volunteer accordingly.

This committee could be a powerful force within a community and a congregation, helping create relationships among people who might not otherwise be involved in one another's lives, and creating opportunities for personal sharing, deeper understanding, and growth.

The committee could take on the responsibility of outreach to people who are homebound and make arrangements for inclusion of homebound people in congregational events, holiday observances and Shabbat services.

25. Prepare Holiday and Shabbat Gift Baskets

Holidays and Shabbat can be lonely times. Brighten up the holidays for people living with AIDS by preparing special baskets of gifts for them for the holidays, or for Shabbat. The basket can contain special foods for the holiday (apples and honey for Rosh ha-Shanah, *hamantashen* for Purim, matzah and macaroons for Passover, etc.), a bottle of grape juice (alcohol doesn't mix with many of the drugs people living with AIDS are taking), or other appropriate items for the holiday, like candles and a _hanukkiyah_ for Hanukkah.

In preparing the baskets, use your creativity and your resources. In every congregation there are people who have businesses that make things. Find out who produces what, and get them to donate items that could be fun or useful for people living with AIDS. Printers put out calendars and notepads all the time.[5] People in craft businesses have all kinds of useful items you could get. You never know what kind of free items you could stuff in these baskets until you start asking for donations.

Always include in the baskets your good wishes for health, strength and healing. Include some of the prayers from this book or others, as well as prayers appropriate for the holiday.

---

[5] I once bought a Louise Hay calendar for a Christmas gift for a friend who was in pretty poor shape. It felt strange buying a calendar for someone who might not live for the year. I didn't know why it was the right gift until I game it to her, and told her I was confident that she would use every last page in it. She did. It was a nice blessing for us both.

Section 4: Shituf B'tsaar: Alleviating Another's Pain

No one wants to suffer alone. And no one wants to hear someone kvetch all the time. But when we participate in improving the life of someone who is suffering, we remove some of the pain, we help lighten the load.

"All Israel is responsible for one another" means that we are always responsible—not only when times are good, and not only for people who are well. Our responsibility for one another includes times when our brothers and sisters are enduring hardships. The commitment of responsibility is not limited in any way. It's not that all Jews who are righteous are responsible for one another, or that all Jews who practice their Judaism in like ways are responsible for one another, or that all Shabbat-observant Jews are responsible for one another. If we are truly responsible for one another, helping people living with AIDS is clearly one way through which we can show our responsibility. Joining in the suffering, and alleviating it, is taking that responsibility seriously.

Leviticus Rabbah 4:6 puts it rather succinctly in two ways: (1) When an animal is beaten on its head or one of its flanks, the whole animal feels it. So it is with Israel. When one of us is hit (or in pain), all of us feel it.[6] (2) People are sitting in a boat. One takes out an awl and starts boring a hole under his seat. His companions say to him: "What are you doing?" He says to them, "What business is it of yours? I'm only boring the hole under *my* seat!"

---

[6] There's a great episode of the original *Star Trek*, in which Spock is stricken with an intense pain. It's almost indescribable to him. He "feels" the deaths of thousands of Vulcans who are killed in one instant. All Vulcans telepathically feel such pain when their people are hurt. Spock reflects on why humans see the horror of the loss of hundreds of lives as more significant, in some way, than the loss of each life. Each loss is painful to a Vulcan.

We are all in the same boat. We all feel the same pain when one of us is ill, or at least we should. The Talmud, *Brakhot* 5b, relates the story of Rabbi Yohanan, who visits Rabbi Hiyyah Bar Abba, who is ill. Rabbi Yohanan simply says, "Give me your hand." Hiyyah gives him his hand, and he "is raised" (he felt better or was cured). Then Rabbi Yohanan gets sick, and Rabbi Hanina comes to visit him. The Talmud asks why he didn't cure himself, as he had done with Rabbi Hiyyah. The Talmud replies that "a prisoner can't free himself." Whether he was a great healer or not, Rabbi Yohanan couldn't cure himself—it takes other people to help alleviate our pain and make us feel better.

It is up to all of us to follow the examples of these rabbis and to help alleviate the pain and sufferings of others—they can't do it all for themselves, and they need our help to free themselves of the burdens of illness, suffering, depression and loneliness.

---------- *Psalm 126: 5-6* --

They who sow in tears will reap with songs of joy.
Though they go along weeping carrying the seed bag,
they shall come back with songs of joy,
carrying sheaves.

26. Host a Dinner for People Living with AIDS and Their Families, Loved Ones and Friends

Community dinners are great vehicles for getting AIDS services and programs going in your community. They require little up-front work, provide opportunities for all kinds of participation, and give people living with AIDS a true sense of community.

A community dinner creates community. By inviting people living with AIDS and their families, friends, and loved ones to a dinner hosted by and involving members of your congregation, you enable people living with AIDS to enter into your community, share time with people who are not so totally wrapped up in surviving AIDS, and begin to develop caring relationships and an "extended family." These dinners will also allow members of your congregation to meet people from other walks of life whom they might not have gotten to meet otherwise. Stereotypes and prejudice are fought by meeting reality.

These dinners are helpful for people living with AIDS, but they also help create community for the caretakers, families, and loved ones who are caring for a person living with AIDS. Dinners give caretakers and friends an opportunity to talk, share experiences, learn from one another, and draw support from others in the congregation. People in the congregation, at the same time, learn about the challenges faced by the caretakers and may volunteer to lend a hand in the caretaking process.

To host a dinner, set a date and time for the dinner, with about eight weeks of planning time. Sunday evenings are good, since few organized activities would be in conflict. But beware: If you are planning your first dinner to take place in the midst of winter, you may not get a lot of participants. If you want to start with caretakers and family, winter is fine, since they might need to get out for a little while.

Finding people interested in coming is a challenge. Put articles and/or advertisements in the local newspapers, post flyers at local hospitals and clinics, contact AIDS service provider organizations in the local area and invite them to send representatives from their staffs and to bring as many clients and friends as they would like. (Since you are not asking for names, they might feel inclined to bring clients.) Contact the family services offices in your community and ask them to post flyers as well. Contact other congregations and invite them to join in your effort, and ask them to post your flyers and announce your event from the pulpit.

Even with all of these efforts, you may get just a few people connected with AIDS at your first event. Don't despair and don't give up. The chief form of communication for many people connected with AIDS is word of mouth. Once you break into the community by demonstrating that your program is good, the food is good, and the community welcoming, they will come. (If you build it...)

Note that you do not want to label people. If people come whom you do not know (in other words, not members of your congregation) don't ask if they are living with AIDS, or if they are a friend, lover, or family member of such a person. They will self-identify, if they want to. Welcoming them means letting them feel comfortable and not on the spot. Everyone should get name tags and use first names only. Do not make any distinction between name tags of members of your congregation and other guests; be sure to get members of the congregation to sit with people they do not know. There's nothing worse than setting up one of these dinners and having all of the congregants sit together while all of the "strangers" sit with one another. This is a guarantee that no one will come back.

The dinner can be potluck or home cooked. If there are people living with AIDS attending, plan a high-calorie, low-fat menu. (This is one of the challenges of living with AIDS. Lots of calories, but digesting fats is a problem. Pastas, proteins, carbohydrates, cooked vegetables are all good.) If you can, find out about any specific dietary needs of people who let you know they're coming, and meet those needs, whatever they are.

Plan a program for after dinner. It can be just about anything, but it's preferable for it to be light and entertaining—Maybe someone who can sing oldies, or a good storyteller. Include in the program blessings and prayers for renewed strength and healing for people who are ill and prayers on behalf of the people who are caring for a loved one who is ill. Samples of such prayers can be found in # 27.

27. Pray/Meditate with People Living with AIDS

When you visit, it is often very helpful to pray or to meditate with a person who is ill. Always ask the person who is ill if it is okay for you to offer a prayer for his or her renewed strength and healing, and invite the person to join you in the prayers if the answer is affirmative. The words, though important, are not as significant as the message that it is okay to pray, to ask for help from a Higher Power, and to do so both alone and together. It is also a good way of leading into discussions that will be very meaningful both for the person who is ill and for the visitor. Prayer can be used to help calm a person and to introduce the idea of meditations for healing and inner peace.

There's a really beautiful note on prayer in *Brakhot* 13a: "The Holy One seems to be far away, but nothing is nearer than God. Let a person pray in an undertone, and God will hear that person's prayer. It is as if one whispers one's thoughts in the ear of a friend. Can you have a God nearer than this, who is as near to people as the mouth to an ear?" [7]

There are a lot of sources you could use for prayers. I have attached just a few prayers. Keep a collection of them; you never know which will fit a particular situation. Whenever possible, pray both for the individual and for all others who are ill. This allows the person who is ill to continue to hope for others as well as for him or herself. Even if one's personal prayers are answered in ways other than one hopes for, if one prays for others, perhaps those prayers will be answered.

---

[7] *The Talmud Anthology:* Louis Newman, p. 341.

Isaiah 54:10

For the mountains may move,
And the hills be shaken,
But My loyalty shall never move from you,
Nor My covenant of friendship be shaken,
Said Adonai, who takes you back in love.

Mi Shebeirach

Mi shebeirach a-vo-tei-nu
M'kor ha-b'ra-cha l'i-mo-tei-nu,
May the Source of Strength
Who blessed the ones before us,
Help us find the courage
To make our lives a blessing,
And let us say, Amen.

Mi shebeirach i-mo-tei-nu
M'kor ha-b'ra-chah l'a-vo-tei-nu,
Bless those in need of healing
With r'fu-a sh'lei-ma,
The renewal of body,
The renewal of spirit,
And let us say, Amen.

(Debbie Friedman and Drorah Setel)

May the One Who blessed our ancestors, Sarah and Abraham, Rebecca and Isaac, Rachel, Leah and Jacob, Moses, Miriam and Aaron, bless and heal _(name)_ and all others touched by AIDS and related illness. Mercifully restore (him/her) to health and vigor. Grant insight to all those who bring healing, courage and faith to _(name)_. Grant love and strength to us and to all who love a person living with AIDS. God, let Your Holy spirit rest upon all who are ill and comfort them. Speedily and soon, may we know a time of complete healing, a healing of body and spirit, and let us say: Amen.

(My translation)

⤳

Eternal God, near to all who call upon You, be with _(name)_ as (s/he) combats AIDS; strengthen (her/his) faith in Your compassion. Grant (her/him) strength and courage to endure suffering and discomfort, and vision to see beyond the present moment. May it be Your will to bring (her/him) peace and healing even as (s/he) journeys through life with AIDS. Grant courage and wisdom to all who minister to (her/his) needs; may their hope and determination never wane. Heal us, Adonai, and we will be healed; save us and we will be saved, for You are our hope and our strength. Amen.

(Author unknown)

⤳

El nah, refah nah lah (lo). God, please, heal her (him).

(Moses said this to God when Miriam was afflicted with leprosy. It's short and to the point.)

(Numbers 12:13)

⤳

Source of Life, we pray You:

Heal them.

Grant courage to those whose bodies, holy proof of Your creative goodness, are violated by the illness, pain and suffering of AIDS.

Heal them.

Grant strength and compassion to families and friends who give their loving care and support, and help them not to despair.

Heal them.

Grant wisdom to those who probe the deepest complexities of Your world, as they labor in the search for treatments and cures.

Heal them.

Grant clarity of vision and strength of purpose to the men and women entrusted with the responsibility for institutions and whole communities. Let them not be swayed by fear and hatred, but let them remember that their greatest obligations are to those least capable of being heard.

Heal them.

Grant insight to us all to understand that whenever death comes, we must accept it—but that before it comes, we must resist it, not only by prolonging life, but by making life truly worthy as long as it is lived.

Heal them and heal us all soon, in our own time, with the ultimate world-healing. Amen.

(Author unknown)

❧

Heal us, Adonai, and we shall be healed. Save us, and we shall be saved. For You are our Praise. Send us complete healing for all of our illnesses, for You are our Nurturant and Loyal Source and Healer. You are a fountain of blessings, Adonai, Who heals the sick.

(Rabbi Marcia Prager)

❧

My God,
The life and soul which You placed within me are pure.
You breathed of Yourself into my flesh,
creating and forming in me a deep awareness of Your presence.
It is You who constantly arouse the desire to live within me.
Sometimes You take this hope from me,
only to renew it again and again,
that I may once more praise You my God and God of my people.
You are the origin of all that happens,
and every soul is a part of You.
Praised are You, Adonai,
constantly renewing life within me,
with Your breath of love.

(Translator unknown)

We are loved by an unending love.
We are embraced by arms that find us
even when we are hidden from ourselves.
We are touched by fingers that soothe us
even when we are too proud for soothing.
We are counseled by voices that guide us
even when we are too embittered to hear.
We are loved by an unending love.

We are supported by hands that uplift us
even in the midst of a fall.
We are urged on by eyes that meet us
even when we are too weak for meeting.
We are loved by an unending love.

Embraced, touched, soothed, and counseled
ours are the arms, the fingers, the voices;
ours are the hands, the eyes, the smiles;
We are loved by an unending love.

(Rabbi Rami Shapiro)

May you live to see your words fulfilled
May your destiny be for worlds still to come
And may you trust in generations past
and yet to be.
May your heart be filled with intuition
and your words be filled with insight.
May songs of praise ever be upon your tongue
and your vision be a straight path before you.
May your eyes shine with the light of holy words
and your face reflect
the brightness of the heavens.

(Talmud *B'rachot* 17A, translated by Rabbi Marcia Prager)

Prayer is powerful and gives strength. I have found, when visiting people who are ill, that they are very ready, willing and interested in having prayers said with and for them. Often people will tell me they don't believe in God, or don't believe in a God who responds to personal prayers, but what could it hurt? (In other words, an opening.) If praying becomes an invitation to discuss the issues of life and death, hope and healing, God and God's love, then it serves its purpose.

Meditation with a person living with AIDS can also be very helpful (to both participants). If nothing else, meditation can bring a calm, a quiet to a person whose life is everything but. Boring as it may be, life in a hospital is far from calming, relaxing, or healing. There are a lot of really good source materials for meditating with a person living with AIDS, so I would suggest you get any of the following sources:

The AIDS Book: Creating a Positive Approach, Louise Hay
The Color of Light, Perry Tilleraas
Healing Visualizations, Gerald Epstein
Heart Thoughts, Louise Hay
Jewish Meditation, Aryeh Kaplan
Peace, Love and Healing, Bernie Siegel
The Power is Within You, Louise Hay

Louise Hay's works are extremely helpful. She has also produced a number of excellent audiotapes for people to listen to and meditate with, as Bernie Siegel has also done. Using these tapes to reinforce your personal meditations with a person living with AIDS can be very helpful.

When Rabbi Glazer first called me, he told me that Richard was in the hospital, looked like he was going to die soon, and he (Rabbi Glazer) could not do that journey with him. So I started to visit Richard. He wasn't ready to die at that time, so we began doing healing meditations to calm him and bring him some peace from his pain. Richard told me his favorite place in the world was a beach in Spain. So we meditated with him visualizing himself on that beach, using the waves to bring in calm, peacefulness and healing and to remove from his body pain, disease, anxiety, fear, and other negative thoughts.

At my third visit Richard looked a little better, and I noticed that he was no longer hooked to an IV bag. So after we meditated I stopped by the nurses' station. I was looking for some kind of confirmation that he was making progress. I had not stopped at the nurse's station before, and they did not know who I was or what I was doing with Richard. I asked, "How is my friend Richard doing?" There were three nurses. One looked up and said, "Well, you know, he has AIDS." So now I knew more about her than about Richard. Another looked up and said, "I think he's doing better. I went in there this morning, I looked at him, and I told him he looked like he was at the beach."

You just never know.

28. Arrange for Services of Comfort and Hope

A service of comfort and hope can have many forms. It can be a part of a special event program, a special, separate worship service, or a regular worship service with a special emphasis on comfort and hope. Its structure depends on the event, circumstances, and timing of the service.

A service of comfort and hope is *not* a segregated service only for people living with AIDS and their caregivers. It should be developed so they can attend but should also involve all of the other members of the congregation, who are the comforters and the hopers for the entire community. It makes a difference to a person living with AIDS to come and worship with an entire community that is concerned for his or her survival and well-being. For this reason it might be preferable that it be a regularly-scheduled worship service with a special emphasis on AIDS.

Services of comfort and hope are also perfect times for dedication of panels to the AIDS Memorial Quilt, as well as good times to acknowledge volunteer efforts.

The actual service should incorporate a prayer for healing for people living with AIDS, a prayer for the strength and well-being of caregivers, a prayer of memory, a prayer of hope, and a statement of commitment. Use prayers listed in #27, as well as the following prayers. Feel free to change them or replace them.

And then all that has divided us will merge
And then all compassion will be wedded to power
And then softness will come to a world that is harsh and unkind
And then both men and women will be gentle
And then both women and men will be strong
And then no person will be subject to another's will
And then all will be rich and free and varied
And then the greed of some will give way to the needs of many
And then all will share equally in the earth's abundance
And then all will care for the sick and the weak and the old
And then all will nourish the young
And then all will cherish life's creatures
And then all will live in harmony with each other and the earth
And then everywhere will be called Eden once again.

(Judy Chicago)

At the rising of the sun and at its going down,
We remember them.

At the blowing of the wind and in the chill of winter,
We remember them.

At the opening of the buds and in the rebirth of spring,
We remember them.

At the shining of the sun and in the warmth of summer,
We remember them.

At the rustling of the leaves and in the beauty of autumn,
We remember them.

At the beginning of the year and at its end,
We remember them.

As long as we live, they too will live;
For they are now a part of us,
As we remember them.

When we are weary and in need of strength,
We remember them.

When we are lost and sick at heart,
We remember them.

When we have joy we yearn to share,
We remember them.

When we have decisions that are difficult to make,
We remember them.

When we have achievements that are based on theirs,
We remember them.

As long as we live, they too will live;
For they are now a part of us,
As we remember them.

(Sylvia Kamens and Jack Reimer)

'Tis a fearful thing
To love
What death can touch
To love, to hope, to dream,
And oh, to lose.
A thing for fools, this,
But a holy thing,
a holy thing to love.

For your life has lived in me,
Your laugh once lifted me,
your word was a gift to me.

To remember this brings painful joy.

'Tis a human thing, love,
A holy thing, to love,
What death has touched.

(Rabbi Chaim Stern)

⸞⸟

El Malei Raḥamim

O God, full of compassion, You who dwell on high, grant perfect rest in Your sheltering presence to all whom we mourn who have died of AIDS. Source of mercy, let them find refuge in the shadow of Your wings, and may their souls be bound up in the bond of eternity. May You be their hope and their possession. May they rest in peace, and let us say, Amen.

⸞⸟

For caregivers:

May the Holy One, who blessed and led our ancestors, bless the care-givers of those who are ill. May they be filled with fortitude and courage, and endowed with sympathy and compassion, as they give strength to those at their side. May they fight against despair and continue to find within themselves the will to reach out to those in need. In their care for others, may they know the blessings of community and faith in each hour of their labor.

In the hour of pain and fatigue, help us to find strength in our hearts. In time of fear and suffering, renew within us the calm spirit of trust and peace. Grant insight to those who bring healing, courage and faith to those who are sick, love and strength to us and to all who love them. God, give strength to Your people. God, bless Your people with peace.

29. Incorporate Prayers for People Living with AIDS into Congregational Services and Events

How relevant can a worship service be today, in the midst of a worsening AIDS crisis, if the word "AIDS" is never once mentioned or even referred to in any prayers during the service? When were prayers on behalf of the ill more necessary? When would be a better time to show that we stand together in this crisis?

Incorporate AIDS into every service at least once, either in connection with a special prayer for healing for all people who are ill, or by using any of the prayers from the service of comfort and hope. It doesn't have to be a big deal, but it will have a big impact and will once again show that God, your congregation, and your community stand firmly on the side of healing and peace. Offering prayers on behalf of the sick, including people living with AIDS, provides members of the congregation with opportunities for their own personal healing, and a chance to stand with their community in their concern and worry.

I participated in a service at a Jewish educators' conference run by "politically correct" people who were very sensitive to the special needs of the deaf. But nowhere during their two Shabbat services was there any mention of healing for the sick, or opportunities for people to express their hopes, grief, fear, or personal prayers. I left wondering whether "politically" correct "meant bereft of spirit or personal meaning"

30. Become a Funding Partner of an AIDS Service Provider.

Few AIDS service providers have enough money to survive. In the days of shrinking federal, state and local budgets, funding for anything but essential emergency services is almost nonexistent. Major foundations have not responded with enough dollars for agencies that serve people living with AIDS, and when they do respond, funding is limited to new or experimental programs. Foundations like to fund temporary programs, and they expect that ongoing funding for programs will come from other sources.

Corporations are often willing to give of their products or services but do not readily lend their names or support to local AIDS service agencies. They almost never provide substantial funds for ongoing programs. The hardest funds to raise are the funds to pay the ongoing salaries of the professional and support staff. United Way and other philanthropic organizations that distribute funds in the local community (like Jewish Federations) are having a lot of trouble raising funds for their long-term programs, and many have had to cut back, making them unable to respond to new needs of people living with AIDS in the local communities.

Given the difficulty in raising funds from the traditional sources, one of the things you and your congregation could do that would be of tremendous help to an AIDS service provider would be to help them raise funds. That way, they can focus their efforts on providing the services that are needed (which is, after all, why they are in business), and you can enable them to do their jobs. By becoming a funding partner you do the fund-raisers (concerts, art auctions, testimonial dinners, whatever); you will have a tremendous impact on your partner agency and the undying gratitude of all the people the agency serves.

I had to resign from my position as Associate Executive Director of the AIDS Interfaith Network because I couldn't afford to continue to work full time and not be paid. When I left, I was owed nearly $25,000 in back salary. (How I survived for 6 months without being paid is a good question.) The irony was that our agency was finally on its way to having some real funding. In my year and a half at the Network, we had increased annual revenues from $35,000 to just over $125,000 when I left. But much of the funding was for specific programs and services. We were able to buy the computers we so desperately needed, the phone system, and the copier with funds from grants. We could get grants for programs, but no one wanted to fund staff. How do you run programs without staff?

Collecting Things for People Living with AIDS

INTRODUCTION: People living with AIDS are often completely penniless just a few months after their first opportunistic infection. Those people who had jobs are no longer working. Once they are not working, they lose their access to health insurance. To qualify for Medicaid, a person has to have almost no money and no assets.

The best way to understand AIDS poverty is to look at an example of what can happen. In 1991, I had pneumonia. I immediately began to worry that it was AIDS related. (It wasn't. Relax.) Instead of lying around, I began worrying. What if it was AIDS? I would be fired from my job, because I would not be able to do it if I was sick. In New Jersey and most other states it is legal to dismiss an employee because of illness. I had about two weeks of sick leave on which I could count. Once I lost my job, I would lose my health insurance. The federal government requires insurance to be continued up to 18 months, but the employee has to pay for it. I called my insurance company. It would cost me $321 monthly to continue my health insurance. The insurance company could drop coverage at any time if they saw indications that the illness was AIDS. *Insurance can be cancelled due to illness.*

I had no disability insurance (and if I had AIDS, I would never be able to get disability coverage). To make matters worse, I own a townhouse in northern New Jersey, which I bought in June of 1987, four months before the real estate market collapsed. In 1991, it was worth exactly $40,000 *less* than I had paid, so I had no savings and no equity. Without a job, sick and with no income to pay my mortgage, maintenance fees, or health insurance coverage, how long would I last? I figured I had 90 days before I was totally bankrupt, unless, of course, I had to be hospitalized. If I were in the hospital, it would end all hope of financial survival upon discharge. I could see myself as a homeless person in 90 days! *In New Jersey more than 50% of people living with AIDS are homeless,* not because they're bums, but because there is no way for them to survive financially. Many live on the generosity of family and friends or kindly strangers with an extra room, basement, or garage.

Once a person living with AIDS hits the financial disaster they have to achieve in order to qualify for Medicaid, he or she can then use the absurdly overcrowded clinics and get minimal health care. (One hospital in Newark has over 2,000 people on the Infectious Disease rolls, and two doctors. Think about the implications that has for their health care!) The bankrupt and certifiably poor and disabled person living with AIDS can then also qualify for Social Security Disability Income, which is based on a fraction of what they were earning when they became disabled. I would have had about $600 monthly for all my expenses: rent, food, transportation, clothing, medications, everything. And remember, I had a good job. My monthly disability income would have been considered high.

If, after a person living with AIDS hits rock bottom financially, he or she becomes hospitalized for a month or two, he or she loses what little he or she may have left. Many people are released from hospitals directly to the streets, the shelters, or the kind of near-homelessness they left when they were hospitalized. So if they actually get into subsidized apartments or rooms somewhere, they have none of the personal or household supplies they need, and they cannot afford to purchase them. I have heard many stories about this total poverty, but none so horrible as that of the person to whom we delivered a box of canned food only to see the person start to cry because he did not have the money to buy a can opener.

Obviously, people living with AIDS need help if they are going to survive. But I would have hesitated to take money from strangers, and I doubt that others feel comfortable living on charity. So your help with supplying the things people living with AIDS need could make a real and meaningful difference in their lives. Ways 31 through 34 tell you what's needed and why.

The person who lengthens the life of a poor person has his or her own life lengthened when his or her time to die arrives. (Zohar iii, 85a)

The life of a person is not true if that person does not take care to help other people in need. (Betzah, 32.)

31. Collect Food for People Living with AIDS

I f you or your congregation are not involved in a food bank, please consider collecting canned and packaged foods for people living with AIDS.[8] Focus on easy-to-cook food with high nutritional content, preferably low in salt and fat but high in calories. Cans and packaged foods last a long time, which may be helpful as you develop a distribution system. Fresh produce, breads, milk products and meats would be great, but first you have to be able to come up with a sure way to get them into the hands of the people who need them *before* they spoil. The following is a list of suggestions of some of the kinds of foods you might collect. It's far from exhaustive. The best rule is, if you'd buy it for yourself, if you find it tasty and nutritious, it's okay to buy it for a person living with AIDS.

Canned vegetables	Canned fruit
Canned and bottled juices and drinks	Macaroni and cheese
Ensure or other dietary supplement drinks	Instant breakfast drinks (they're easy to make and can be used all day)
Brand-name cereals	Canned meals (Spaghetti O's, Cup o' crackers (all kinds) Noodles, or similar)
Herbal teas	Rice-a-Roni meals in a box
Fruit rolls/ fruit snacks	Canned or dry soups and bouillon (avoid high-sodium soups)
Nuts	Hot cereals, like oatmeal, in single-serving packets
Cookies	Coffee (ground and instant)
Rice (all kinds)	Hot chocolate in single-serving packets
Beans (all kinds)	Sugar, salt, pepper, other spices

---

[8] (If you are involved with a food bank, please continue to support it as you have always done. Food banks serve all kinds of needy people who depend on you for support. Look at "Ways" 32 through 34 for other projects you can undertake.)

Jell-O & instant pudding

Raisins

Canned tuna (in water)

Dry packaged pasta and bottles of pasta sauce

Peanut butter, jellies and jams

Please do *not* collect:

Spam (too much salt and fat)

Canned pumpkin or cranberry sauce (Usually donated to food banks in the spring, when everyone cleans out their cabinets. What does a person living with AIDS need 10 cans of pumpkin or cranberry sauce for? Collect necessary, quality foods.)

Dinty Moore products or similar (Too much salt and fat. Hidden message is this is cheap stuff for rich people to buy for poor people. Not the message you want to give.)

Canned asparagus (Who eats that stuff, anyway?)

Anything that will not keep on shelves for a month or more

Home canned items

Out-of-date or opened packages

32. Collect Over-the-Counter Medications and Personal Hygiene Products

O ver-the-counter medications are a particular problem for people living with AIDS. Many can't be accessed through Medicaid, which pays for prescription medications only. Food stamps do not pay for medications. So simple items like Tylenol or Pepto Bismol are difficult for people living with AIDS to obtain. One method for raising people's awareness of this problem and getting them to help is to encourage people to buy two over-the-counter products whenever they buy one for themselves. Set a collection date every six weeks.

The following list is a sampling of some of the products people living with AIDS need your help in getting:

Tylenol	Buffered aspirin
Antacids	Cold and flu remedies (nonalcoholic)
Cough drops	Antihistamines
Preparation H or similar	Pepto Bismol or similar
ImmOdium or similar	Laxatives
Band-Aids	Hydrogen peroxide
Betadine	Epsom salts
Antiseptic creams	Vicks Vapo-Rub or similar
Visine	Monistat 7 or similar[9]

Vitamins (multis, C, D, iron, E, minerals, etc.)

Skin creams and anti-itch lotions (hydrocortisone creams)

---

[9] The FDA made these products for vaginal yeast infections nonprescription, which is terrific for most women. But the number one symptom for women with AIDS is chronic vaginal infections. Now that these products are nonprescription, they are not covered by Medicaid. They are also extremely expensive.

Personal Hygiene Products:

Toothpaste (preferably for sensitive teeth and gums or Mentadent)[10]

Toothbrushes[11]	Dental floss
Mouthwash	Shampoo (hypoallergenic)
Soap (hypoallergenic)[12]	Deodorants
Talcum powders and antifungal powders	Tampons and sanitary napkins
Combs and brushes	Shaving cream
Disposable razors	Kleenex
Condoms[13]	Washcloths and hand towels

I asked the South Orange, N.J., Clergy Association to collect any one item on our list. They insisted I choose which item would be most useful. I decided on vitamins. So they put out their newsletters, and in many of the congregations in South Orange, on a specific date, vitamins were collected to help people living with AIDS. It was an ordinary collection, a few hundred bottles of assorted vitamins.

About two months later, I got a call from the executive director of one of the congregations. She was a little concerned because one of her members was sending in vitamins, and it would take more than a car to get them from the synagogue to our office. I told her we'd take two cars. She called a little later and said it might still be too much for two cars. I suggested that she have the person supplying the vitamins bring them directly to our office, instead of the synagogue. I gave her directions to get to the office.

About an hour later an 18-wheel tractor trailer pulled up and started unloading! The packing list had a total value of $10,450 **wholesale!** *A member of one of the congregations makes the bottles that vitamins go in. He called three of his customers, who donated these vitamins. You never know.*

---

[10] People living with AIDS often have very sensitive gums and sores in their mouths. Toothpaste for sensitive teeth enables them to brush and maintain their teeth even with their gum problems. The only dental care they can get through Medicaid is extractions.

[11] One symptom of AIDS is oral thrush, a fungus in the mouth. It can be treated and prevented by using a new toothbrush every week and using a toothpaste with no sugar. Hydrogen peroxide and baking soda toothpaste is best for this condition, but toothpaste for sensitive teeth is also helpful.

[12] People living with AIDS get all kinds of skin irritations and rashes. Hypoallergenic soaps and shampoos can help.

[13] Some people living with AIDS are sexually active. Condoms are expensive.

33. Collect Household Supplies for People Living with AIDS.

I f you can barely afford to pay for food, buying simple household supplies becomes a real challenge. People living with AIDS need to live in an environment that won't make them sick, yet they may not be able to afford to buy the very items that can help them keep the germs to a minimum. They also need to be able to prepare meals, which means they need basic kitchen equipment.

Basic Kitchen Equipment

Frying pan	1- and 2-quart pots with covers
Kitchen towels	Potholders
Can opener	Wooden spoons
Spatula and pot stirrer	Sponges
Rubber gloves (the thick ones, to wash dishes and pots and pans)	
Mixing bowls	Measuring cups and spoons

Basic Household Cleaning Equipment

Sponges	Paper towels
Dishwashing liquid	Rubber gloves (the heavy-duty kind for scrubbing)
Bleach	Laundry detergent (free of scents and unnecessary chemicals)
Bathroom cleaners	Dryer fabric softeners (scent-free)
Mop, broom & dustpan, pail	All-purpose cleansers (like Mr. Clean)
Toilet paper and tissues	Toilet inserts (2000 Flushes or similar)

34. Collect Clothing for People Living with AIDS

People living with AIDS often do not have the money to buy new clothing, and as the disease progresses, the size of their clothing changes repeatedly. Many women living with AIDS are also mothers who have to clothe their children (who may also have AIDS), and all of these clothes can be very expensive for people on a limited budget.

Many AIDS service provider organizations are aware of the great need for clothing for people living with AIDS but do not have the people to organize, or the space to store, a clothes bank. It's very hard to get high-quality used clothing that is clean, in good condition, immediately usable (correct season), easily identified and sorted by size, and useful to people living with AIDS. (Few people living with AIDS have a real need for blazers and ties, formal or fancy wear, etc.)

There are two ways you can help with clothing: Establish either a clothing bank or a "Raid the Closet" program.

•

A. Clothing Bank

A clothing bank is a place where clothes are collected, sorted, organized and stored for distribution to people living with AIDS. The clothes could be donated by a special drive throughout the congregation or community, with the specification that you are looking for certain kinds of clothing, as noted above (no formal wear, correct season, clean, in good condition, etc.). Be prepared to have all kinds of unacceptable clothing donated by well-meaning people who don't understand that this is not just a convenient way of cleaning out their closets. Have a plan for what you will do with the clothing you can't distribute.

Once you get the clothing, sort it by size and type so you have some idea of what you have, and display it in some way. Then let AIDS service providers know that you have a clothes bank for people living with AIDS, and invite them to bring their clients and participants to the bank. Transportation might be a problem, so try to come up with a plan for how you will cope. (Buses from agencies, carpools, and volunteers are all good options.)

Be sure that the clothes bank reflects the values of caring for people living with AIDS at every step of its implementation. If it's open only at specific times and days, be sure they are when public transportation is available, and on dates that do not conflict with major community events or ongoing programs. (For instance, if your community has a daily lunch program for people living with AIDS, it would not be a good idea to have the times of your clothes bank limited to 11:00-1:00 daily.) Make it a welcoming environment, with something to drink and eat available for anyone who comes for clothing, and be sure to post information about any other programs or events in a prominent area.

B. "Raid the Closet."

Collect and sort the clothing as above, but arrange with AIDS service provider organizations for you to bring the collection to display and to give away at that AIDS service provider's site. Schedule a date, have a bunch of your own volunteers on hand to help people find things they want and need, bring refreshments, and have a "Raid the Closet" party. Be sure to bring bags or some other means for people to carry their "new" clothes home.

Once you get either of these programs going, it should be relatively easy to get new clothing and shoes donated by department stores and clothing stores, which often throw away unsold and out-of-style clothing and shoes. Check your local malls and see what ends up in the dumpsters. You'll be shocked. The stores will not give you anything unless you can prove that all merchandise will go to an ongoing distribution program for people living with AIDS, so your program has to be ongoing first. The other limitation for this idea is that you will get precisely the kinds of clothing the stores couldn't sell at any price. On the other hand, if you have someone in your congregation or community in the wholesale garment business, who knows what kinds of things you can get?

A variation on this idea is a "Raid the Linen Closet" event for towels, sheets, pillowcases, place mats, etc.

35. Develop a Plan for Distribution of the Supplies Collected in 31-34 Above.

Nothing collected for a person living with AIDS does any good until it is in the hands of the person for whom it was collected. The last thing you want to do is develop a full warehouse. Before you start collecting, figure out how people living with AIDS are going to get what you are collecting. There are two options: They can come to you, or you can go to them. The question is how.

If you work with an AIDS service provider organization whose clients come regularly to an office, or one that delivers items or meals to people living with AIDS, you can dovetail your plans with their distribution systems. This method is the easiest, because it involves only bringing the collected items to the office and letting the service provider distribute them. If clients come to the office regularly, find out what the busiest day is, and designate that as the day you will give out whatever you are collecting to anyone who wants it. (It's not your job to determine eligibility or any other qualification. If you're distributing oral hygiene products, give them to everyone who wants them. If you are distributing at an AIDS service provider organization, everyone who comes in the door is, in some way, connected with a person living with AIDS. Remember, confidentiality is important. You are not there to invade the privacy of people living with AIDS.)

If you are not working with an AIDS service provider organization, distribution will be a lot harder. You could work by referral from hospitals and social service workers, but understand that you are not providing case management services; anyone the social workers refer to you is qualified by the social worker's referral.

If you are planning to develop a delivery system using volunteers, this is an excellent opportunity to train the volunteers in being sensitive to the needs of the people they will see on their routes. Make sure they know all the facts and myths about AIDS and are on the lookout for unmet needs at the homes of people they are visiting.

36. Think About How the Things You or Your Company Use or Make; Can Be of Use to People Living with AIDS or to AIDS Service Providers ....

It seems almost obvious, but many people never think about donating some of the very items they make or sell for a living. If you're in a business that makes anything, can it be used by or for people living with AIDS? Similarly, if it can't be used in any way, do any of the people you buy from, or who buy from you, make items that could be of use to people living with AIDS? If the answer to any of these questions is yes, see how you can be of help by contacting an AIDS service provider organization.

The item may even be something that can help an organization, and thus, indirectly, the people living with AIDS we all want to help. Used office furniture, computers and office equipment could be just what an agency needs but cannot afford to buy. (We received a donation of two suites of office furniture from a major corporation that was closing down a regional office. The furniture was much more extravagant than we could have imagined, and in perfect condition. The corporation didn't make anything we could use, but one of their staff people was thinking creatively.) The donations could also be something that would help in a fund-raising event, such as bottled water, soft drinks and fruit for a walk-a-thon, door prizes for an event or awards for helpful volunteers.

In North Jersey we have a program that distributes a teddy bear or stuffed animal to every person they know living with AIDS, young and old. We also have the world's largest manufacturer of stuffed animals right here in North Jersey. Does anyone know anyone who could authorize the ongoing donation of stuffed animals by this company?

37. Visit a Display of the AIDS Memorial Quilt, or Arrange for a Display

The AIDS Memorial Quilt has been displayed in its entirety only twice in Washington, and in smaller pieces throughout the United States. There are now over 25,000 panels included in the Quilt, and it continues to grow. (Over 200,000 people have died of AIDS-related causes, so it may continue to grow for a long time to come.) The quilt is a remarkable memorial, horrible and wonderful at the same time. It's odd for a memorial to be built as a crisis continues, but part of the mission of the Quilt is to provide support for local AIDS programs, and help prevent additional deaths due to AIDS. Visit the Quilt when it's in your town, or bring panels for display in your town if it is not scheduled in your area. To contact the national office of the Names Project: The AIDS Memorial Quilt, call 415-882-5500. Ask if there is a local chapter serving your area. If there is, contact the local chapter and ask them to provide you with a display. If there is no local chapter, discuss a display with the people at the national office.

When I visited the AIDS Memorial Quilt in Washington, D.C., in October of 1992, I was overwhelmed by the experience. It had been a rainy morning, so the quilt was late in being opened. All around its perimeter there were thousands of people waiting to enter into the Quilt. I walked through this crowd, because I was alone, and because there was nothing else to do. I walked to an area where new panels were being placed that had just been dedicated to the quilt during this weekend. There were thousands of them. All new. And unlike the rest of the panels, which are sewn together in groups, these were all separate. I walked down aisle after aisle of new panels, reading name after name after name, seeing lives reflected in color and design.

As I walked among the panels for the dead, speakers began reading names of people who had died of AIDS. I was overcome with a feeling that was horrible and yet familiar. It was the same feeling I have when I walk through Yad Vashem in Jerusalem, the memorial for the six million Jews who were murdered in the Holocaust. Just as the names in Yad Vashem (literally a Memorial and a Name) called out to me, reflecting the overwhelming devastation of so many lives, the names on the panels of the Quilt were calling out to me. I was hearing the echoes of one holocaust in the midst of another.

38. Create a Panel for the Quilt

I f you knew someone who died of AIDS, has a panel been made for him or her? If not, make one. Or you can make a panel for people from your congregation or community who have died of AIDS-related causes, or for a group of people who have died. You can get a list of people who have died from local AIDS service providers, who often need help memorializing people with whom they have worked. Making a panel is an act of memory, of love and of commitment not to forget the people we have lost.

For information about how to make a panel, contact your local chapter of the Names Project or the national office at 415-882-5500.

Basically, the panel has to be a rectangle of 3 feet by 6 feet, with at least 6 inches extra all around for it to be bound to the other panels in the Quilt. It can be made of any kind of material, but you will want to use something sturdy, like sailcloth or denim. All items attached to the panel should be sewed on, not glued or pasted, since panels are folded and opened often, and glue will not hold under the conditions the panel will be put through. You can use any materials you choose for decorating the panel; once again, keep in mind that what you use should last (glitter will come off almost immediately). The message on your panel should reflect the life and loves of the person you are remembering. Many include the full name of the person and his or her dates of birth and death.

Panels do not have to be done alone. Some of the best "grief work" a family, friends or a community can do in mourning their loss can be done together in designing and creating a panel. Gather the loved ones together, and together plan and sew the panel.

Psalm 21: 5-7

They asked You for life; You granted it; long life, everlasting.
Great is their glory through Your victory; You have endowed them with
  splendor and majesty.
You have made them blessed forever, gladdened them with the joy of
  Your presence.

39. Say Kaddish for People Who Have Died of AIDS

The Union of American Hebrew Congregations designed a panel for the AIDS Memorial Quilt that says "Who will say kaddish for me?" Too many people have died of AIDS with no loved ones or family to say kaddish for them. When there is no one to say kaddish, it means that there is no one who is regularly remembering the person who died. Take responsibility for saying kaddish for someone who has died of AIDS, whether you actually knew the person well or not. While I would not want anyone's recognition of AIDS to revolve exclusively around death, a lot of people have already died of AIDS. It's up to us to preserve their memories.

If you are leading services, note in announcing kaddish that you are saying kaddish for people who have died of AIDS who have no one else to say kaddish for them. Your statement of support and commitment will not go unnoticed in your congregation.

At *Yizkor* services, invite people who are not remembering immediate relatives to stay with the congregation and to say *Yizkor* for people who have died of AIDS and have no one to remember them. (Both of these ways of remembering are done for people who died in the Holocaust. Perhaps the invitation should be for people to say *Yizkor* for people who have died in either the Holocaust or of AIDS, or who have no one left to say it for them.)

Ecclesiastes 7:1

A good name is better than fragrant oil, and the day of death better than the day of birth.

40. Develop a Transportation System for People Living with AIDS ...

People living with AIDS often become unable to drive themselves anywhere for numerous reasons. Many have to "cash in" their cars and can't afford to drive. People who have problems with their vision, brain lesions that could cause seizures, or other kinds of neurological problems are not allowed to drive, even though their problems may occur extremely infrequently.

Public transportation might be a solution for them if they live in a city, and if public transportation is good and the routes are extensive. In northern New Jersey, that is not the case. Anyone living in the suburbs (or even in the cities) faces real challenges using public transportation, which is extremely slow, costly, and not designed for people with a chronic disease. Waiting at bus stops in rain, snow, or cold temperatures is not a good idea for a person who has no immune system. The lengthy ride, the wait and lack of restroom facilities is also a major problem, since many people living with AIDS have a need for regular visits to restrooms. Routes and schedules are designed for business commuting, not necessarily for access to clinics or hospitals. Some areas are simply not accessible by public transportation.

To develop a system to help people living with AIDS with transportation to doctors' offices, supermarkets, support group meetings, clinics, etc., recruit people who have cars and are willing to give a few hours weekly to help people in need. Contact an AIDS service provider organization, and let them know you have volunteers who would like to assist people with transportation. As requests for help come in, assign drivers. When requests are for transportation to attend meetings of support groups or workshops for people living with AIDS, and people need rides from several locations that are relatively close together, be sure to maximize your volunteers by having each one pick up more than one person. If the volunteers are going to wait to bring their passengers home, be sure that they are invited in by the AIDS service provider agency and treated well, as any volunteer should be. Perhaps the agency has some envelopes to be stuffed or some other work the volunteer can do while he or she waits (no one likes to be unproductive).

41. Invite People Living with AIDS to Holiday and Shabbat Events ...

Many non-Jewish communities do a great job of reaching out to people in need, particularly for Thanksgiving and Christmas. Congregational parties often have some connection with giving charity—either needy people are invited to the event, or things are collected at the event to be given to people in need afterward. Christmas parties are often set up by outreach committees for other organizations that serve people in need.

Yet many people need more than just a one-shot fix of welcoming community each year. Develop a plan for involving people living with AIDS, both mobile and homebound, in all of your congregation's events. If your congregation has a special meal for a certain holiday, make sure people living with AIDS are personally and specifically invited to come to the meal, free of charge. (Of course, no one else should know the identities of the people living with AIDS or that they did not pay for the meal. Confidentiality is really important here. No one wants to be labeled "poor" or "sick." If they choose to self-identify, that's fine, but it's also their choice.) If your congregation has other special events, like a Purim or Hanukkah party, or a Tikkun for Shavuot, reach out and invite people living with AIDS to participate.

Passover Seders are excellent opportunities to reach out and make a difference in the lifes of people living with AIDS—and in the lives of their families and friends. Ask a few families to invite people living with AIDS to come to their Seders, and arrange transportation for these guests. Many people living with AIDS feel very isolated from their own families and may not have anyplace to go for this event. An invitation to your Seder may be precisely what a person needs to come back into being a member of your community.

42. Take Care of a Child of a Person Living with AIDS

People living with AIDS often can't handle all of the demands of their lives. Some parents living with AIDS are not able to do all of the day-to-day family management chores. For instance, getting children up and ready for school may be an overwhelming task; preparing meals for children may be too much. Be a volunteer to help get the kids out of the house a few days a week, or to help make dinner for the family a few days weekly.

The children who have a chronically-ill parent may also need some special attention. Big Brother/Big Sister organizations exist in many areas and help children whose home life is difficult. However, not all parents living with AIDS have signed their children up to participate in these kinds of programs, and they may not be available in all locations.

Encourage parents living with AIDS to enroll their children in Big Brother/Big Sister programs, and become active in such a program yourself. If an agency is available in your area, it is best to use the agency structure for establishing the Big Brother/Big Sister relationship, rather than doing it informally on your own. The agency will have a training program, supervision and activities that will help you as a volunteer. The agency will also be available to assist you should there be any problems or misunderstandings. In addition, the agency will continue looking out for the welfare of the child if you get sick, leave town, or have to take on some other kind of project. It will also find additional ways of helping the parent if necessary.

If no Big Brother/Big Sister organization exists in your area, consider volunteering to help develop a program for children of people living with AIDS through an AIDS service provider organization. Many organizations do not touch on this need because they already have their professional hands full. If you will volunteer to get the program going, and develop it so it does not cost anything or is self-funding, you might be able to turn a possibility into a reality and have a tremendous impact on the next generation of people whose lives are touched by AIDS.

Section 5: Tikkun Olam: Make the World a Better Place

W hen God created the world, it was left incomplete. God's intention and expectation was for people to complete the job of creation, to be partners in making the world a whole, perfect place for people and animals. In Genesis 2:5, God provides rain, but people have to till the soil. Creation included and culminated with people. Our mission on earth is bringing wholeness, *sh'leimut*, the complete quality of peace, to the world. Beyond tilling and maintaining the earth, we are supposed to go on to better the world, perfecting it. This is called *tikkun olam*, repairing the world.

God is the ultimate role model of lovingkindness. In *Sotah* 14a, Rabbi Simlai states that the Torah begins with an act of lovingkindness: God clothes the first people of creation. The Torah ends with an act of lovingkindness: God buries Moses. It is in these kinds of deeds that people are supposed to imitate God, who clothes the naked, cares for the oppressed, visits the sick, comforts mourners, buries the dead, is merciful and gracious to all people. We learn from this that no one should think of him or herself as too good or too important for the humblest forms of human help and sympathy. To walk humbly with God (Micah 6:8) means walking with God in funeral processions, wedding processions, marches and protests on behalf of people who are suffering, and everything in between.[14]

Isaiah affirms that though God wants ritual Jewish behavior, such as observance of Shabbat, the most important demand God makes of people concerns the ways in which we take care of each other, acting in God-like ways:

---

[14] Based on excerpts from *The Talmud Anthology* by Louis Newman, pp.152-3.

Is such the fast I desire,
A day for people to starve their bodies?
Is it bowing the head like a bulrush
And lying in sackcloth and ashes?
Do you call that a fast,
A day when Adonai is favorable?
No, this is the fast I desire:
To unlock the fetters of wickedness,
And untie the cords of lawlessness,
To let the oppressed go free;
To break off every yoke.
It is to share your bread with the hungry,
And to take the wretched poor into your home;
When you see the naked, to clothe them,
And not to ignore your own kin. (Isaiah 58:5-6)

Acts of lovingkindness, of caring for other people, of respect and dignity for all people, even the oppressed, even the naked, are what God demands of us. Nowhere in Isaiah's words do we find room for people to sit in judgment of other people for their situations. Nowhere does Isaiah say that we should care for only certain groups of people in need. Doing God's work on earth, as God's partners in completing creation, requires that we act like God, loving and caring for all people.

Hillel taught: "If I am not for myself, who will be? If I am only for myself, what am I? If not now, when?" This applies to the AIDS epidemic as well. We have to be concerned not only for ourselves but for all other people, no matter what they are living with—and we can't put off the help we are supposed to offer. We have to be reasonable about self-protection, reducing the spread of AIDS, and providing appropriate AIDS prevention education. But at the same time, if all we do is worry about how AIDS might affect people who are not infected, what are we? AIDS prevention educational programs are an important *start.* But if they are *all* we do, what are we?

If we sit back in complacency and watch as people die and lives are ruined, we are just being selfish. Whether or not we are personally confronted by people in our lives with AIDS, we are obligated to reach out to others in crisis. It is precisely for this reason that AIDS is a religious issue and should involve people from all Jewish communities, from Reform to Orthodox. All of us are obligated to help, without any reservations. Hillel never implies that his questions apply only to specific groups of people whom we like more than others for some reason.

AIDS is a holocaust of a different time. "In Germany they first came for the Communists and I didn't speak up because I wasn't a Communist. Then they came for the Jews, and I didn't speak up because I wasn't a Jew. Then they came for the trade unionists, and I didn't speak up because I wasn't a trade unionist. Then they came for the Catholics and I didn't speak up because I was a Protestant. Then they came for me and by that time no one was left to speak up."[15] HIV/AIDS has had a similar progression, first affecting Haitians and gays, then intravenous drug users and heterosexuals in Africa, now teenage women in the United States.[16] When do we decide to speak up? When no one else is left?

Jews have had a long tradition of involvement in social justice issues and causes throughout the ages. We are commanded to remember that we were slaves in Egypt, and that we must work for the freedom and well-being of others precisely because we have had this experience as a people. *Tikkun olam*, repairing the world, includes improving the lives of people living with AIDS, looking out for their needs and their rights.

Tzedek, tzedek, tirdof: Justice, justice you must pursue.
Deuteronomy 16:20

---

[15] Pastor Martin Niemoller

[16] *The Record*, March 14, 1994. A Northern New Jersey newspaper reported the latest statistics of gloom. New AIDS infections up 111% in 1993. Fastest growing population of new infections: women in their late teens and early 20's.

43. Arrange to Deliver Hot Meals to Homebound People Living with AIDS

There are two basic ways of getting hot meals to people living with AIDS: (1) prepare food for them and deliver it, or (2) get donations of meals from local restaurants and deliver them. If you can get a few people together to cook meals on a regular basis, and to deliver the meals while they are still hot, this would be a tremendous help to homebound people living with AIDS. All the visits they may get, even the people they have shopping for them or taking care of their household needs, may not address the need for a good meal and the good wishes that come with it. One of the best fund-raising letters I have ever read was from God's Love We Deliver, which provides hot meals daily to people living with AIDS. The letter described one of their typical clients, who was very grateful to his "buddy" volunteer who had done the shopping for him but cried after the buddy left because he didn't have the strength to cook the food.

Cooking meals for people living with AIDS gives them more than food; it makes it very clear that someone is out there caring for them, literally feeding them their concern and care (See #15 above). If people already receive a meal from an AIDS service provider organization, it's easy to get that organization to help with distribution, and the extra meal will be deeply appreciated. If there is no program available in your local community, your delivery of hot meals will be even more deeply appreciated. To identify people in need, contact local AIDS service provider organizations, and tell them you will deliver hot meals to homebound people living with AIDS on a regular basis. They should be able to give you a list of people who need this help after they get the permission of their clients.

The other idea, getting food donated by local restaurants, makes the lives of volunteers easier and gets even more people involved. Every restaurant has leftovers. Many restaurants throw away entire meals that are still good, that they can't sell. Either on an individual basis or as a group, you can get volunteers who frequent local restaurants to speak with their owners or managers and establish a day and time that is convenient for pickup of leftover meals. Make sure the restaurant owner or manager knows that the meals are for people living with AIDS, so he or she can feel good about being involved in helping. They will package a meal, just as they would do a "doggy bag" for a cutomer, with appropriate serving containers. If one volunteer gets one meal from one restaurant and delivers it to one person, it's a very non-demanding job for the volunteers, makes it easy for the restaurant to oblige, and will make a real difference in the life of one person. To meet additional needs, just get more volunteers to do the driving, and recruit the participation of more restaurants. You'll need one person to coordinate the project if it involves more than one place.

Be sure to appropriately acknowledge the help of the restaurants. A nice certificate suitable for framing, which could be hung somewhere in the restaurant, will go a long way to foster good relations and continuing generosity.

44. Cook Special Meals for People Living with AIDS in Group Homes

People living with AIDS in group homes also need some special attention. No matter the size of the group home or the quality of the cooking staff, a special meal prepared by a group of volunteers (or, in a small group home, by an individual) for the people in the home is always deeply appreciated. It allows for some variety, a change of pace and a change of taste. It creates opportunities for meeting and becoming involved with other people, and opportunities for real sharing and breaking down barriers. Some group homes for people living with AIDS are very small; some are larger. Depending on the homes in you community, develop a plan to provide one special meal monthly for the residents, allowing volunteers to meet and share dinner with residents of the home.

In Essex County, NJ, the only residential facility for homeless people living with AIDS is Broughton House, which provides transitional housing for up to six months and helps homeless people find places to live by the end of that time. Numerous churches bring a monthly meal for the residents and their families and friends, and volunteers attend these meals. I have attended a few times when one congregation, the Glen Ridge Congregational Church, was providing the meals. It's a wonderful sight: relatively wealthy women from a suburban church talking and sharing with people from minority backgrounds who are living with AIDS. Many establish ongoing relationships with the residents, and the church (as well as individuals) regularly helps people through the transition to their own apartments with furniture, household equipment, and the things they need to get their lives together. The support for the individuals and for the residence is exemplary of what can come from just making a meal once a month for people living with AIDS.

If there is a group home in your community, offer to bring a dinner. They won't turn you down. (Check if there are any special dietary requirements, and meet them.)

45. Develop an Unrestricted Fund for Emergencies

People living with AIDS and their families often experience all kinds of financial emergencies, such as special medical needs that Medicaid or insurance will not cover, funeral expenses (Children of mothers living with AIDS also die. Imagine the stress and nightmare of losing a child and not being able to pay the funeral expenses!), temporary room and board expenses, household expenses (like heat) that are out of control, etc.

The list of emergency needs is unlimited. A mother needed to go to California to be with her dying son, but could not afford airfare. We couldn't help her and could find no agency that could. The government has no agency for helping with family emergencies like this. How do impoverished people pay for funerals, emergency airfare, or other urgent situations?

I worked with a person who had just come from a drug rehabilitation program, had no money, no job, no place to stay, no clothes other than what was on his back, and no hope for any change in the near future. I called the welfare office. They told me he would be eligible to go to a shelter (where he would probably be raped). To get financial help from welfare, he would have to bring in a pay stub. When I explained that he was not working and that was why he needed welfare, I was informed that he, therefore, would not qualify for welfare. He could get $144 monthly in emergency funds in two weeks. What he was to do in the meantime was not welfare's problem. I paid his living expenses out of my own pocket for the month and found a few ministers with discretionary funds to help.

Creation of an unrestricted emergency fund would have a tremendous impact on emergency needs. Allocation of funds should be handled by a very small confidential committee that meets quickly and reachrs decisions *very quickly.* Just a few hundred dollars in unrestricted emergency funds could make a meaningful difference in an emergency. The mother who had to get to California needed just $350 for airfare. The recovering drug addict needed about $200. Abuse is possible, but unlikely. People tend to respect this kind of goodwill and help. Funds can be replenished by fund-raisers and donations.

46. Provide Special Programs for Professional Caregivers

AIDS affects all kinds of people in many different ways. Professional caregivers for people living with AIDS live with incredibly intense pressure and stress. Hospital and clinic workers often experience the worst of the disease; they only see people living with AIDS when they are in greatest need of attention. Agonizing deaths are constant, as are what may seem to be hopeless and painful treatments. Social workers experience unending crisis and frustration along the path through the maze of government and agency bureaucracies. The professional turnover and burnout in these agencies is tremendous, even with good group work and careful planning.

Caring for the people who are professionally involved can have a tremendous impact on their spirits, which in turn can have a positive effect on the lives of the people for whom they care. I have three suggestions for how you can make it possible. Sometimes we do not thank people who are paid, because they are just doing their jobs. But no one is ever paid enough for the kind of work professionals do for people living with AIDS. If we want people to go above and beyond the call of duty and their basic responsibilities, then we should recognize their efforts.

1. Host a dinner for AIDS professionals who work at a local hospitals, clinics and agencies. Contact the head social workers from each program, inform them of your desire to host a dinner for professionals at your congregation, and get their help in planning the dinner. Develop some form of entertainment or programming that is light and enjoyable. (I would advise against a lecture on AIDS or health care; let them have a break.) Include in the programming some form of spiritual healing, such as prayers on their behalf, for people who are ill,

and in memory of people who have died in their care. Give them all something that says thank you to take home, to put on their desks, to look at when they need it. You can get children involved in the program by having them make "thank you drawings" or art projects for this purpose. Anything you can think of to say thank you will be deeply appreciated.

This dinner will provide a special break for the caregiving professionals and give them opportunities for sharing their experiences informally, networking and finding new allies in their local community.

2. Facilitate making a panel for the AIDS Memorial Quilt with professionals from local agencies or hospitals. They have all been in constant contact with the dead and the dying. How are they memorializing the people they have lost? How are they expressing their grief? Help them make a panel for the people who have come through their agencies' doors, and involve everyone in the process of creating the panel. It can have hundreds of names on it, or just a few. The process is the important part, but the panel will symbolize the process of mourning the losses every caring professional feels in this epidemic.

3. Develop other ways of recognizing the humanity of people who are caring for the people living with AIDS. A picture wall, with the pictures and names and statements from all of the caring people who have worked or are still working in the agency, can send the message that people are important and appreciated. The picture wall could also serve as a client wall. Develop an area for the pictures of all of the people who use the services of the agency or program. The juxtaposition of the two—professionals and the people they serve—can help everyone who enters to see the humanity and partnership of both parties in the healing process.

4. Adopt an agency. Provide a home-cooked meal for AIDS professionals at an agency once a month. As with providing a meal for people living with AIDS, this meal could be prepared by members of a local congregation and delivered, served and joined in by members of the congregation, who share the meal, hear what's going on, and can become friends of the caring professionals. It's a relatively easy

process but can give a tremendous boost to their spirits and their sense of not being alone.

I met with the Chief of Infectious Diseases at a local inner-city hospital when we were both part of a panel on caring for people living with AIDS. He was clearly dedicated to the task and cared deeply about his patients. But he was also very depressed. He kept talking about the fact that most of his patients die, and there is nothing he can do about it. He said repeatedly that most of his patients were "goners." What kinds of messages was he giving his patients?

47. Provide Space for AIDS Service Providers to Hold Support Group Meetings or Leadership Meetings

Space is often difficult to come by. But meetings in convenient places are necessary for agencies and programs to function. As was mentioned above, many AIDS service provider organizations work on a very tight budget and cannot afford to pay rent to outside organizations for meeting space. If your building is open and space is available, allow AIDS service providers to use the space free of charge. Many AIDS service providers have offices in cities but need to be able to reach out to clients and donors in the suburbs. Making space available for them would be most appreciated.

Making space available also enables people in your congregation to have the opportunity to connect with the program or service being offered, and perhaps to become more involved in the work of that program or service.

48. Help Facilitate Support Groups for Unmet Needs

What needs are not being met in your community? How do you find out?

Call an AIDS service provider and ask. They will gladly tell you what is needed and what is not needed. Consider reaching out to provide services that are desperately needed but that are not areas of major focus for service providers, who are worrying about survival needs of their clients. The following are samples, not an exhaustive list, of unmet needs:

1. **Bereavement groups** for the survivors of people who lived with AIDS. Bereavement groups are available in most communities but often involve people who have lost loved ones to all kinds of causes. The survivors of people who died of AIDS are different and often do not feel that they fit in with general bereavement groups. While grief is grief and the needs of the bereaved are the same, whether we like it or not, AIDS phobia, homophobia, and issues that have nothing to do with bereavement often block the involvement of the survivors of AIDS deaths in general bereavement groups. Even in death it may be difficult for people to talk about losing the battle with AIDS and the possible discrimination they now face.

   Unfortunately, AIDS bereavement groups are becoming more and more necessary.

2. **Primary caretaker support** is both a major challenge and a great need. People who become the primary caretakers for people living with AIDS often neglect all else in their lives to care for the person living with AIDS who is ill. They live with the incredible stress of

both helping a loved one in anguish and watching that person die a slow and painful death. Primary caretakers deserve medals for what they do. They give life, prolong life, and ease suffering.

However, instead of getting medals, many lose their jobs, feel abandoned by their families and friends, are extremely lonely and isolated, and often ultimately lose the loved one they have cared for so tenderly.

Support groups are a possibility for caretakers, if they can come. But note that they have almost as little control over their day-to-day lives as the people who are ill. Regular support group meetings should take place during the early evening, when it might be possible to arrange for someone else to be with the person who is ill.

However, it might be more helpful to focus the energy of the group toward a training program of some kind, such as studying about nutrition for people who are wasting, or new medical techniques, or meditation techniques for the chronically ill. Primary caretakers will be more inclined to come to meetings if they can come away with something concrete they can *do* to help their loved ones. While we know they need opportunities to talk and to express their feelings, primary caretakers may not see the value in a support group. They *will* see the value in a training program, and then the support becomes a subtle, important by-product.

3. **Training groups for the "worried well."** People who are HIV positive, who are not ill, and who want to stay that way need specific training programs in nutrition, vitamins, exercise, stress reduction techniques, meditation techniques and new medical procedures for maintaining their health. Not enough research has been done on why people who are HIV positive become ill with AIDS or stay healthy. Every community needs to focus energy on keeping people well, yet few are doing this lifesaving job. Training programs for the "worried well" have the potential to save lives. Once again, support group sessions for people who are well might work, but they will probably not be well attended. Make them practical, with things people can do to stay well, and they will come. The support is automatic in the group and will happen as a by-product of the training.

4. **Training for people who are living with AIDS.** When a person is living with AIDS he or she is not always unable to get out of the house. Many people living with AIDS are mobile and well enough to work, to go to group meetings and programs. Training programs for people living with AIDS can be extremely helpful to them. For instance, assertiveness training can be helpful for people who have never before had to negotiate with the entitlement systems, or training programs can help people to take control of their medical care. The numbers and kinds of programs are limited only by the talents, abilities, and interests of the people organizing the training programs.

Consider establishing an ongoing training program for people living with AIDS. Some possible programs are T'ai Chi movement classes, spirituality, meditation and relaxation techniques, vitamins and nutrition, latest clinical research, music and art therapy, etc. For many of these programs speakers and teachers can be found free of charge, or, if you need funding, hold special fund-raisers. For one class once a week, with little or no overhead, it's not going to be all that expensive. Just don't build a new agency around these programs.

5. **Mothers who have lost a child of any age to AIDS.** While I know it may seem sexist, mothers are often very different from fathers in their experience of a loss. In our society men go on, hide their emotions, and have heart attacks or strokes. Mothers cope with the pain of the loss of a child in very different ways. Once again, while they might not come to support group meetings to "cry" as a group, they will often come together for a task-oriented project or ongoing program. Women who were the primary caretakers for their children and experienced the deaths of their children alone or with minimal support from their families or husbands might be willing to serve as "buddies" for other mothers who are going through the experience. Others might be interested in learning how to be political activists in local, state and national arenas. Still others might be interested in reaching out to AIDS services providers to create other forms of support, including developing financial help for agencies.

Mothers are an incredibly powerful lobbying force, a force to be reckoned with in the service-provider community, and a tremendous support for others who are going through the same experiences. Mothers who have lost a children need each other, and they need a goal to work toward, to channel their grief, their anger, and their energies in constructive directions.

Tapping in to this strength is a double benefit; it can dramatically change the face of AIDS in a local community as it provides support and comfort for people whose grief will never end. Find some mothers by asking AIDS service providers who is out there; invite them to a meeting; do some brainstorming together as to what is needed and what they are interested in doing; develop outreach components for involvement of other mothers; and they will go places no man has gone before.

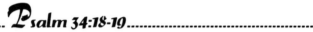

Psalm 34:18-19

They cry out, and Adonai hears,
and saves them from all troubles.
Adonai is close to the brokenhearted;
those crushed in spirit God delivers.

49. Lead Letter-Writing Campaigns to Politicians

Political activism works. But after more than 13 years of this epidemic, the people who have been leading the political activism need some support; it's time to bring in the reserves. Politicians look for all kinds of trends in their mail and phone calls. A religious group is often noticed, particularly when it comes to AIDS or other issues where the conservative right has proven effective. Politicians need to be made aware that there are other religiously-committed people out there who want to see more services, programs, research, and funding for the needs of people living with AIDS. When they only hear from one group of people, they tend to think the vocal ones are representative of the feelings and ideas of their entire community.

Develop a political action team to monitor political action in your local community and state. Establish connections with one of the national political action groups as well, so you can support their efforts on a national level. Once you have people looking at what is going on politically, begin to respond to issues as they arise with letters, phone calls and personal meetings.

If nothing is on the legislative agenda directly relating to AIDS, it may be up to you to deal with the legislative gap. There isn't a state in the union that doesn't have to deal with issues relating to the treatment and care of people living with AIDS.

50. Give of Yourself— Your Own Talents and Professional Abilities.

Even if you don't have the time for a lot of volunteer work, giving of your professional talents may make a huge difference to each individual you help. No matter what you do—doctor, dentist, lawyer, accountant, therapist, hair cutter—if you provide a service to people, there are people living with AIDS who need your help. Call an AIDS service provider organization and let them know you are available for one or two clients per month (or week or day) free of charge. They will refer people to you as soon as they hear of the need for your service. (If they don't, contact another agency.)

51. Give Money.

General donations: This should be obvious, but sometimes we lose track of the fact that agencies need financial support. Sometimes we get so many mail appeals that we chuck them all immediately into the trash. No matter how you feel about mail appeals, give. If you're not very committed to a specific program or service, give to them all. *If you have a favorite, don't give till it hurts; give till it feels good.*

We are obligated to give *tzedakah* (charity) to the needy. But the word *tzedakah* is rooted in the word *tzedek.* "Justice giving" is not a handout; it is an enactment of justice.

Your dollars make a huge difference. Agencies cannot function without the ongoing support of donors.

We have all heard about charities where the funds do not go for the purposes intended. This is a serious problem for all of the very worthy and responsible charities in our communities. It's very easy to check on what a charity does with your money. Ask for an annual report or a budget. Look at the listing of the board of directors, and see if there is anyone you know. Talk to the staff people. Just don't make them go nuts for a donation of less than $18. It's not worth their time.

The vast majority of charities whose mailings you will get are both legitimate and providing essential services for people living with AIDS. If you prefer to give to a program or service with which you are familiar, go visit a local AIDS service provider. Just remember, though, that when you visit you are taking essential time of a staff person who should be focusing on helping people living with AIDS. A lengthy visit for a small donation is not fair to the agency or to the people it serves.

Try budgeting funds for an AIDS service provider once a month, and send a donation out whenever your pay your bills. If you can afford a donation of $18 or more once a month, and let the agency know you will be sending it to them every month, they know they can count on you and your $216 (or more) annually. That's roughly 60 cents daily, less than a cup of coffee or a phone call in New Jersey. It makes a real difference.

Memorial Donations: One of the realities with which we live is that many people living with AIDS die. When that happens it can bring comfort to the family, loved ones, and community to honor the memory of the deceased by establishing a memorial fund at an AIDS service provider organization. Ask that people make donations to this memorial fund after the funeral, during and after the *shiva* mourning period, and at other times when people gather in memory of the deceased, and give them pre-addressed envelopes to make the process easier. If possible, leave the fund an unrestricted one for the agency to use in any way it needs, so the money actually gets put to use. The last thing we need to do in a time of crisis is establish ongoing endowment funds with the agency able to use only a fraction of the funds donated. If the agency has a specific project that can be named in memory of the deceased, that's great. But do not limit the agency in this way if you can avoid it. The point of the memorial fund is to use it to help as many people as possible as soon as possible in memory of the person who has died.

Memorial funds can also be replenished each year as the survivors mark the anniversary of the death of the person, or the birthday, or other significant dates.

52. Include Funds for People Living with AIDS in Your Celebrations

We all have reasons to celebrate. But we are all in the middle of a crisis. While we take time out of the struggle of living to celebrate the blessings in our lives, we also have to be aware of the needs of other people who are not celebrating with us. We may want to invite them to join in the party, or we may want to have a more lasting impact on their lives. I have two party suggestions:

1. While you celebrate, help others survive. When you plan your party, figure out what it will cost you and take a percentage of that amount to give to an AIDS service provider organization. You'll hardly miss the extra percentage. If the government were taxing your party at 6%, you'd pay it. Let people living with AIDS tax your party.

2. Do you really need the gifts you're going to get? At my last housewarming party I got a lot of wine (I don't drink any alcohol), lots of stupid gifts (like green potholders in the shape of fish), and a few too-expensive items that made me wonder about the rationality of the giver. I would have been much happier with gifts that meant something.

Put on your invitation an indication that gifts are not necessary. But if people are inclined to give a gift, let them know that the most appreciated gift would be a meaningful donation to the charity of your choice. List a few choices, with a description of what each charity does and the mailing address. Gifts in honor of a happy occasion are most welcome at AIDS service provider agencies, which rarely get to participate in any way in celebrations. They also enable the agency to expand its mailing list to include all of the people who give in your honor, so they can be encouraged to continue giving in the future.

3. Thank you gifts. We often give party favors at the end of parties. In your bag of cookies, include a note that a donation has been made to an AIDS service provider organization by you in honor of your guests. Invite them to send additional donations if they enjoyed the party. Include the address and a brief description of the work the agency does.

53. Make Holidays More Spiritually Meaningful with Special Donations

Holiday parties can be opportunities for sharing support for AIDS service provider organizations. Rather than exchanging gifts, have a charitable donation exchange. Everyone donates the $5 or $10 (or whatever they would have spent on the grab bag gifts) to a charity in honor of someone else. Provide a list of possible charities, including AIDS service providers (though you may want to include other options as well). This idea has a lot of potential to make of gift-giving very spiritually meaningful for all of the participants, who do not really need the grab bag items.

Holiday cards and acknowledgments are available through many AIDS service provider organizations. Instead of investing your money in Hallmark greeting cards, give the money to an AIDS service provider selling holiday greeting cards. Most are reasonably priced and include in the cost of each card a percentage that is donated to the charity. To further personalize your holiday cards, add a red ribbon and the hope that the recipient will wear the ribbon or use it to decorate his or her home during the holidays.

By sending special donation cards, encouraging other people to give to AIDS charities, you will be involving new people in the struggle, showing your support, and having a direct impact on the face of AIDS in your community. In many ways your actions will reflect the values that holidays are supposed to celebrate.

54. Stand Up for the Civil Rights of People Living with AIDS

People living with AIDS not only face a difficult chronic illness, they also face stigma, discrimination, hatred and fear. They may not always have the energy or the time to stand up for their own rights. That's where you can come in.

Go to the protests and marches. Become involved in the political process. Speak up when you hear about the infringement of their rights. Speak up when you hear AIDS jokes, when you hear or see someone being treated unfairly.

As we know all too well, when one group of people is threatened we are all at risk. It is up to us, the people who are well, to look out for the people who are not, just as we would want done for us if we became weak. We can't wait for justice to happen; we have to make it happen.

Budget cuts threaten to deny people living with AIDS the services and programs that have been established for them. Government leadership changes; community priorities change. People who are well are obligated to be on the front lines of the protests, because people who are not well just can't do it themselves, and because they have a right to expect the help of people who believe that justice is everyone's responsibility.

F uture generations will turn to you and will ask, "What did you do to help end the AIDS crisis?" How will you answer them?

This book is just a beginning. Use the ideas included here, or any others you can come up with—I am sure there are more than 54 ways to help people living with AIDS. The important thing to remember is that people are dying out there—we have to act now, to respond actively and with as much effort and care as we can.

Patience is no virtue. According to our tradition, it's the opposite. We are told in *Pirkei Avot* that the work is great, and the time is short. It's not up to us to finish the job, but neither are we free not to get started at it. That's what the starfish story at the beginning of this book is all about. We cannot sit back and be patient. We cannot allow things to be wrong and do nothing about those things but be patient and (maybe) pray. We are commanded: *Tzedek, tzedek tirdof*—Justice, justice you must pursue. We are commanded to correct injustices and to make them right.

We cannot sit back and say we have to be patient when we talk about providing health care to all of the people in this country, young and old, well and ill. We cannot sit idly by and wait patiently for fairness, justice, and equality to come for all of the people of this land. We cannot allow communities to think they have the right to exclude and judge people based on the color of their skin, their gender, their sexual orientation or their illness. If the civil rights of one group can be denied because of who that group is or whom people love, all of our rights are in jeopardy. If a group of right-wing people in Alabama can determine that people living with AIDS have no civil rights, do we wait for them to determine

141

that Jews (or other groups) similarly have no civil rights before we act in response?

We have to make things happen. We have to walk down the paths that lead to justice, even if it's an arduous journey. Getting onto that road, and journeying on that road, is the virtue, not patience. People in need of support of any kind—financial, emotional, spiritual, familial—people in need of healing, a helping hand or a personal touch are our responsibility. We are obligated to make our opinion known and to lend a hand.

Give to *tzedakah*. Pursue justice. Reach out your hand to help. We have no time to waste. We may not have to finish the job, but we certainly do have to get started at bringing justice into the world. Who knows? The justice we pursue today, the *tzedakah* we give, the stand we take, may be precisely what we would want when we or our loved ones are threatened or in need.

---------- *Job 11:17-18* --

Life will be brighter than noon,
You will shine, you will be like the morning.
You will be secure, for there is hope,
And, entrenched, you will rest secure.

.........AIDS Glossary.................................

AIDS—Acquired immunodeficiency syndrome, a complex syndrome characterized by the depletion of the body's immune system, or ability to fight off diseases. AIDS is not a disease in itself, it is a series of opportunistic infections which invade the body as the immune system deteriorates and becomes unable to fend them off.

Alternative therapies—Non-medical treatments of HIV and AIDS, usually natural and nontoxic, which are used to promote healing and to strengthen a person living with AIDS.

Anemia—Many people living with AIDS develop severe anemia, which makes them very tired and weak, as a symptom of AIDS or as a side effect from some of the drugs which they take. Anemia is a depletion of the oxygen-carrying materials of the blood. Treatments include blood transfusions and medical therapies. Iron and mineral supplements may be helpful.

Antibodies to the HIV virus (or any other virus) are cells created by the body's immune system to fight off infections. The presence of antibodies to HIV in a person means that the person with these antibodies has been exposed to HIV and is attempting to fight it off.

Asymptomatic—A person who has antibodies to HIV and does not have opportunistic infections or symptoms of AIDS.

AZT—The first antiviral drug which was believed to retard the progression of AIDS. While still in use, it is not believed to be very effective, and many researchers find it does more harm than good.

CD4 cells or T cells—White blood cells whose function is to fight off infections. Think of the Dow Bathroom Cleaner "scrubbing bubbles." T cells, or CD4 cells, do the same job, they roll through the blood system and scrub out infections. People living with AIDS have fewer and fewer T cells, and therefore cannot fight off infections.

Cryptococcus—Usually a harmless fungus, it causes meningitis in people living with AIDS. Most of the drugs necessary to treat this fungus are extremely toxic.

Cryptosporidiosis— An infection which can cause severe digestive problems for people living with AIDS, including severe diarrhea, dehydration and malnutrition. The infection comes from microscopic protozoa in water and uncooked foods.

Cytomegalovirus (CMV)—An opportunistic infection from the herpes family which attacks the digestive system, the lungs, brain or the retina. CMV is one of the main causes of blindness (and death) among people living with AIDS. This is the infection many people with AIDS fear the most.

Fungus—Tiny organisms which thrive in moist areas of the body. Fungal infections can be found on the feet, in the mouth, sinuses, groin, or in other areas. People with normal immune systems can often fight off most fungal infection.

Hemophilia—A hereditary disease of the blood which prevents it from clotting. Many hemophiliacs require blood transfusions. Prior to 1985, when the blood supply began to be tested for AIDS, many hemophiliacs were infected with HIV by these transfusions.

Hepatitis—An inflammation of the liver which can cause the skin and eyes to yellow. Symptoms can include pain, vomiting, and general ill feeling. Hepatitis can be caused by viral infections and some drugs for AIDS, and can be fatal.

Herpes—The virus which causes cold sores and genital sores. In people with compromised immune systems, herpes has to be medically treated.

HIV (Human Immunodeficiency Virus)—The virus believed to cause AIDS; it depletes and destroys CD4 (T) cells.

Immune system—Cells in the body which protect it from illness. People living with AIDS have "compromised" immune systems, which cannot fight off infections.

ID—Infectious disease. Many hospitals treat people living with AIDS in their infectious disease clinics.

IV drugs—Drugs which are administered through intravenous needles directly into the bloodstream. Heroin, some forms of cocaine and other addictive drugs are abused by people who "shoot up" these drugs directly into their blood systems. When they do not properly clean their needles and share the hypodermic needles with other people, small amounts of blood remain in the needle. This blood then gets inserted into another person. In terms of AIDS, if the blood is HIV infected, this can lead to the infection of another person. The danger of IV drug use is not the drugs, it's the needles. (Drug abuse is clearly not healthy for anyone. But in and of themselves IV drugs are not a risk factor for AIDS. The needles are.)

Kaposi's sarcoma (KS)—A cancer of small blood vessels, first appearing as purple spots on the legs or arms. KS can also invade internal organs such as the lungs. KS seems to be one of the more treatable opportunistic infections and has been decreasing as a cause of death for people living with AIDS.

Lymph nodes—Glands located in the groin, neck, underarms and other locations in the body which filter out microorganisms, fight infections, and produce lymphocytes.

Lymphocytes—White blood cells which fight off viruses and microorganisms.

Mainstream treatments—The medical model utilizing drugs approved by the FDA and prescribed by doctors.

Marinol—The derivative of marijuana which can help improve the appetite, available in perscription form.

Mycobacterium avium intracellulare (MAI)— A form of tuberculosis which invades other organs of the body in addition to, or intead of, the lungs. MAI is particularly difficult to treat after it has spread throughout the body. Prophylactic protocols are being developed; some are successful.

Neuropathies—When opportunistic infections invade the nervous system, neuropathies may develop, limiting the use of hands, fingers, feet and legs.

Pneumocystis carinii pneumonia (PCP)—A pneumonia which is common for people living with AIDS. People with normal immune systems are generally not affected by the parasite pneumocystis carinii. This was once the leading cause of death for people living with AIDS, but prophylactic treatments may prevent infection.

Prophylaxis—Prevention of an opportunistic infection. Some infections, like PCP, can (possibly) be prevented through regular preventative therapy.

Shingles—A painful viral infection of nerve paths on either side of the body. Shingles comes from the same virus as chicken pox (herpes zoster), and in people living with AIDS can be deadly. People living with AIDS who have had chicken pox as children may not be immune to shingles—remember, their immune systems do not work.

"T" cells—See CD4 cells.

Thrush—A fungal infection in the mouth, tongue or throat caused by a candida fungus. People living with AIDS are often infected with thrush, which can be treated with medication, frequent brushing of teeth, gums and tongue with toothpastes which do not contain any sugars, and rinsing with hydrogen peroxide and baking soda. It is important for people with Thrush to change their toothbrushes at least once each week, and to maintain a rigorous oral hygiene schedule.

Toxoplasmosis—An opportunistic infection of the brain caused by the parasite toxoplasma gondii, which is allegedly spread by cats and birds. People living with AIDS should exercise caution in changing the litter box or the cage lining if they have these pets. (Better yet, they should have someone else be responsible for these chores.) (Better yet, they should get a dog.)

Tuberculosis (TB)—A potentially deadly disease caused by tubercle bacillus, a bacteria, which produces lesions in the lungs. It was thought that tuberculosis had been under control, until it recently resurfaced in a drug-resistant form as a major infection among people living with AIDS. Tuberculosis therapies take between nine months and a year to completely rid a person of the bacteria. Drug resistent strains may take even longer. Since tuberculosis is a communicable disease which can be spread in the air to healthy people as well as people living with AIDS, it is very important to regularly test people for TB, to wear masks when working with people who have active TB, and to follow prophylaxis protocols.

Virus—A microscopic organism which is not a complete cell and usually depends on living cells for survival. Viruses cause colds, flus, chicken pox, mumps, etc.

Wasting syndrome—Many people living with AIDS lose the desire or ability to eat or to digest food. Recurrent abdominal pain, diarrhea, dehydration and significant weight loss are often symptoms of the syndrome. Wasting syndrome can be fatal, with people literally starving to death. It can be treated with total parenteral nutrition (TPN) an intravenous therapy, which usually requires overnight use, since it can take up to eight hours to drip. There are significant side effects to long-term TPN use, though. Appetite stimulants, like Megace and Marinol are available, but have to be coupled with therapies for prevention of diarrhea and increased absorption of nutrients. Many people supplement their diets with Ensure or Advera, which are high in calories, proteins and vitamins.

Glossary of Hebrew Terms

Adonai—Literally means "my master," and is traditionally used as a reference to God's name, which we cannot pronounce. I use *Adonai* in translating prayers, even though it is not a translation, since there is no equivalent word in English.

Bar and Bat Mitzvah Ceremonies—Celebrated when a boy turns 13 or a girl 12, these ceremonies mark the beginning of responsibility for a Jewish person. A child who reaches these ages, becomes obligated to fulfill the mitzvot (commandments).

Bikkur Holim—Visiting the sick.

Book of Ecclesiastes—A Biblical book of wisdom, Kohelet (or Ecclesiastes) is a book ascribed to King Solomon which has a particularly cynical outlook.

Brakhot—Blessings

El Malei Rahamim—A prayer asking the God who is full of mercy to have compassion for the soul of a person who is dead.

Hai—Life. The numerical equivalent of the letters in the word hai (*het* and *yud*) is 18. The number 18 and multiples of 18 are seen as special spiritual reminders of life itself.

Hamantashen—Special triangular cookies prepared for the celebration of Purim.

Hannukah—A winter festival lasting for 8 days which celebrates the victory of ancient Hebrews over the forces of Greece. It is celebrated by lighting candles in a special Hanukkah candlabrum, singing songs and eating special Hanukkah foods, like potato latkes (pancakes).

Hanukkiyah—The special candlabrum used for the Hannukah candles.

Hillel—Leading teacher of first-century C.E. Jews in Israel, often involved in controversy with Shammai regarding how to interpret the Oral Law.

Holocaust—The murder of more than six million Jews by the Nazis from 1939-1945 in Eastern Europe.

Kaddish—A prayer which is recited by mourners for eleven months after the death of a loved one, on the anniversary of the death, and during memorial services. The prayer affirms that God's name is great and powerful. It does not mention death, but because it has been recited by mourners for thousands of years, it has taken on a special meaning of comfort for mourners and for the soul in transition or resting in the world to come.

Kvetch—Complain.

Leviticus Rabbah— A book including folklore, stories, law , homiletics and commentaries on the Book of Leviticus from the same time-period as the Mishnah, around 200 B.C.E.

Matzah Balls—Dumplings made from matzah meal which are the essential components of a good bowl of soup.

Mi she-bei-rakh—The first two words of a prayer which begins, "May the One who blessed our ancestors, Abraham and Sarah, Isaac and Rebecca, Jacob and Leah and Rachel, grant a complete a perfect recovery to…"

Migdal Eder—A town in ancient Israel.

Mitzvah—Commandment or good deed. Plural: Mitzvot

Passover Seders—Special meals celebrating the Holiday of Passover. During the meal, the story of the liberation of ancient Jews from slavery in Egypt is told, and songs praising God are sung.

Pikuah Nefesh—Saving lives.

Pirkei Avot—A volume of Rabbinic wisdom literature included in the Talmud.

Psalms—A Biblical book which includes poetry and hymns of praise for God. It is traditional to read Psalms in times of trouble, pain and sorrow as a source of comfort, and at all other times as a source of inspiration.

Purim—A festival celebrating the rescue of ancient Jews from an edict which would have led to their mass execution.

Rosh ha-Shanah—The holiday commemorating the creation of the world, celebrating the new Jewish year. Rosh ha-shanah is the beginning of a period of reflection and self-examination prior to Yom Kippur, the Day of Atonement. On Rosh ha-shanah, it is traditional to eat foods that are round and apples dipped in honey.

Sakanah Hamirah D'asurah—Getting out of danger is more important than observing a commandment not to do something. To protect onself from danger, one can abrogate other commandments.

Shabbat—The seventh day, the day of rest.

Shaddai—One of the names for God.

Shavuot—A festival celebrating the first harvest of the year, 49 days after the second day of Passover. Shavuot commemorates the giving of Torah at Mount Sinai, which completes the process of liberation of the Jewish people from slavery—the laws from God are the guide for how to live in freedom.

Shekhinah—The holy Presence of God. The Shekhinah is considered to reflect the female attributes of God.

Shituf B'tsaar—Participating in the alleviation of someone else's pain.

Talmud—The basis for Jewish law and interpretation of how people are supposed to fulfill God's will. The Talmud contains the "Oral Law", oral traditions which complement and enhance our understanding of Torah. While Judaism is spiritually based on the Bible, Jewish law (halakhah) is based on the discussions included in the Talmud. The Talmud has 36 volumes, called tractates. I have cited quotations from the following tractates: Kiddushin, Nedarim, Sanhedrin, Sotah, Shabbat, Yoma, Derech Eretz.

Talmud Torah—Learning.

Tikkun for Shavuot—An all-night study session on the eve of Shavuot.

Tzedakah—Often mistranslated "charity," tzedakah is the active pursuit of justice. We are commanded to pursue justice, engage in acts of righteousness, it is not an option. Giving to tzedakah—funds to help the needy—is one essential means of pursuit of justice.

Tikkun Olam—Making the world a better place, fixing the world.

Torah—The first five books of the Bible, telling the story of the Jewish people from the beginning of history through the life of Moses. Torah is also a generic word for all Jewish learning.

Tzedek—Justice.

United Jewish Appeal—National Jewish funding organization which provides funds for Jewish needs throughout the world and in Israel. Funds are raised for the UJA by over 200 Jewish federations around the country, providing for both local and overseas needs.

Yizkor—Literally "remember," this word is the opening word of the memorial prayers recited four times annually on Yom Kippur, Shemini Atzeret, Passover and Shavuot.

Yom Kippur—The Day of Atonement, a fast day for confession and forgiveness of sins.

Resource Directories

The following directories will be helpful to you in getting access to more information or learning more in order to directly help people living with AIDS. I have tried to provide you with as much information as I could, recognizing that I could be hunting for resources forever. Depending on what you are planning to do, these lists can point you in the right direction.

The resource directories include a listing of every HOTLINE I could find, in case you need information right now. The listing of agencies and services serves two purposes: (1) Call them if you need specific help for someone, or want more information on what an agency provides, and (2) use the listing to choose an agency, or type of agency, you want to help or to set up in your local community.

You will probably note the lack of agencies which focus exclusively on children and AIDS on this list. This was a conscious choice. Children with AIDS are tragic; the potential loss of any life to AIDS is tragic. *But all people living with AIDS are innocent; no one deserves to get AIDS.* Children with AIDS are a *tiny* percentage of the overall epidemic. Yet some people view the focus on children with AIDS as a "safe" way to help people living with AIDS, so they focus a congregation's or group's efforts exclusively on "innocent" children. This is both misleading and, in my opinion, immoral. The few agencies which focus on children with AIDS do important, heartbreaking and vital work, don't' get me wrong, but they are neither the focus of this book nor real and meaningful responses to the epidemic.

The book resources are divided into four categories: (1) Books on Surviving AIDS, (2) Self-Healing, Meditation and Prayer, (3) Inspiration, and (4) Thinking About *Olam HaBah* (the World to Come). The categories are nice, but there's a lot of crossover from one to another. Once again, remember that this list is not a summary of everything that is available, just what I have read or heard about that fit into the themes of this book and that I thought might be useful. I tried to note what makes each book particularly useful or helpful. There are plenty of other materials out there.

Directories

Many communities have listings of programs, services and resources for people living with AIDS. To get a copy of this kind of directory, call a local AIDS service provider in your area. Many service providers are listed in the phone book under the heading "AIDS," but not all.

The Centers for Disease Control (CDC) has a 24-hour/7 day-a-week hotline for referrals and information. Call them if you need information on programs and services in your area. (But beware, a national clearinghouse is limited. Their information is a start, but may not include all programs and services in your area.) 800-342-AIDS (English) • 800-344-7432 (Spanish) • 800-243-7889 (TDD/deaf Access)

Hotlines

AIDS Clinical Trials Information Service: 800-874-2574

Directory of National Helplines: 800-678-2345

Gaynet: 800-4-GAYNET. (National referral service for gays and lesbians with emotional or substance-abuse issues)

National AIDS Hotline for Hearing Impaired: 800-243-7889

National Hospicelink: 800-331-1620

National Native American AIDS Hotline: 800-283-2437

National Sexually Transmitted Diseases Hotline: 800-227-8922

Project Inform National Hotline: 800-822-7422

TTY/TDD Clinical Trial Hotline: 800-243-7012

Treatment Information and Newsletters

The best method to keep current is to read the newsletters and magazines. Everything changes rapidly with AIDS. New ideas and trends for treatment and for care of people living with AIDS come up often, as do new threats to the civil and human rights of people living with AIDS. All of the magazines and newsletters listed below are useful and informative. Remember, Talmud Torah (learning) includes knowing as much as you can and never becoming complacent with your knowledge.

"AIDS Treatment News", c/o John James, P.O Box 411256, San Francisco, CA (biweekly), 415-255-0588/800-873-2812

American Foundation for AIDS Research (AmFAR), "Treatment Directory," 733 Third Avenue, New York, NY 10017-3204, 1-800-39-AMFAR, ext. 106

"Being Alive/LA" (monthly), 213-667-3262

"The Body Positive" (monthly), 2095 Broadway, Sutie 306, New York, NY 10023, Hotline: 212-721-1346

"Bulletin of Experimental Treatments for AIDS" (BETA), c/o San Francisco AIDS Foundation, 415-863-AIDS

"The Caregiver's Companion", P.O. Box 276, New York, NY 10013, 212-226-0169

"CPS InfoPack" (quarterly), 800-842-0502

"Critical Path AIDS Project" (bimonthly), 215-545-2212

"Notes from the Underground", PWA Health Group, 150 West 26th Street, Rm 201. New York, NY 10001, 212-255-0520

"PI Perspectives Newsletter" from Project Inform, 347 Delores Street, Suite 301, San Francisco, CA 94110, 800-822-7422, California toll free: 800-334-7422, Local: 415-558-9051.

"POZ" published bimonthly Strucbo, Inc., P.O. Box 1279, Old Chelsea Station, New York, NY 10113-1279, 800-883-2163, fax: 212-675-8505. Terrific new magazine for people who are "poz"itive. The magazine includes (among many other things) a listing of buyers clubs and payment assistance programs which may be extremely helpful for people living with AIDS with limited funds. It also includes an "HIV Standard of Care" which is very useful for people who want to be able to take greater and more informed control of their medical care.

"PWA Coalition Newsline" and "SIDAahora" (Spanish/English quarterlies), 50 West 17th Street, 8th Floor, New York, N.Y. 10011, 212-647-1415

"Step Perspectives" (quarterly), 800-869-7837

"Treatment Issues" Gay Men's Health Crisis (GMHC), 129 West 20th Street, New York, N.Y. 10011, Hotline: 212-807-6655, TDD 212-645-7470 (for hearing impaired)

"T & D Digest" (Treatment and data digest of ACT UP/NY), 135 West 29th Street, 10th floor, New York, N.Y. 10001, 212-564-AIDS

Agencies and Services

This list is a start—I have not attempted to list all AIDS service providers in the United States, especially since the list would change so often. I have tried to list agencies which are either unique or which can refer you to a similar agency in other locations, or can answer questions you might have. Being in the New York Metropolitan area, this list includes mainly New York services. Feel free to call them. Also feel free to send them donations—they deserve them!

AIDS Action Council, 202-986-1300. Lobbies for services, funding and programs.

AIDS and Adolescents Network of New York, 121 Sixth Avenue, 6th floor, New York, N.Y. 10013, 212-925-6675. Offers resources, newsletters and resource guides for youth service providers.

AIDS Foundation of Chicago, 312-642-5454. Information, education, referrals.

AIDS Foundation of San Diego, 619-686-5000. Education, support groups, prevention projects.

AIDS National Interfaith Network, 110 Maryland Avenue N.E. Rm 504, Washington, D.C. 20002, 202-546-0807. Counseling, support groups, outreach education, information and policy analysis.

AIDS Pastoral Care Network, 312-334-5333. Publishes a newsletter, referrals for clergy assistance.

AIDS Project Los Angeles (APLA), 1313 North Vine Street, Los Angeles, CA 90028, Hotline: 800-922-2347, Office: 213-962-1600, TDD: 800-553-2347. Wide variety of services for people living with AIDS.

Being Alive 3625 Sunset Blvd., Los Angeles, CA 90026

Body Positive, 236 West 73rd Street, 2nd floor, New York, N.Y. 10023, 212-721-1618. Group counseling, support services and a positive outlook.

Boston AIDS Action Committee., 617-437-6200. Support groups, legal assistance, housing.

Choice in Dying—The National Center for the Right to Die, 250 West 57th Street, New York, NY 10107, 212-586-6248. Offers advocacy and assistance with living wills and proxies. Offers legal counseling for people living with AIDS and their families.

Friends in Deed, 594 Broadway, Suite 706, New York, NY 10012, 212-925-2009.

The Gay and Lesbian Community Service Center of Los Angeles, 1625 N. Hudson, Los Angeles, CA 90028 (213) 933-7400 Goodman Clinic (213) 993-7600—The largest anonymous test site in Los Angeles County. The Center runs the Jeffrey Goodman Clinic full services clinic specializing in AIDS care. Also the center runs Stop AIDS peer education program. CAIN a computerized AIDS Information Network, Legal Services, Counseling, Youth Services and Addiction Recovery services for people with AIDS.

Gay Men's Health Crisis (GMHC), 129 West 20th Street, New York, NY 10011, Hotline: 212-807-6655, TDD: 212-645-7470. Every service under the sun, except spiritual or religious.

God's Love, We Deliver, 895 Amsterdam Avenue, New York, NY 10025, 212-865-4900. Delivers hot, nutritious meals to homebound people living with AIDS.

Healing Alternatives Foundation Treatment and Resource Library, 1748 Market Street, San Francisco, CA 94102, 415-626-4053.

Health Crisis Network, Miami, FL, 305-751-7751. Counseling, education, buddy program.

Health Education AIDS Liaison (HEAL), 16 East 16th Street, New York, NY 10003, 212-674-HOPE (4673). Holistic and alternative treatment and referral information.

Hoffman Center for Holistic Medicine, 40 East 30th Street, New York, NY 10016, 212-779-1744. Nutrition, including herbal and dietary counseling, homeopathy, vitamin and other alternative therapies.

Jewish AIDS Services, 6505 Wilshire Boulevard, #608, Los Angeles, CA 90048 (213) 643-8313 fax (213) 655-1978

Jewish Board of Family and Children's Services, 120 West 57th Street, New York, NY 10019, 212-582-9100. Provides individual counseling, support groups, volunteer training and "friendly visitors," day treatment center and scattered-site housing for people living with AIDS. My friend, Mel Rosen, got this program going, and I am very proud to be serving in his memory as a Rabbinic Intern, running healing circles and other programs at JBFCS. Leah Mason, the department director, is terrific.

The Jewish Healing Center, 141 Alton Avenue, San Francisco, CA 94116, 415-387-4999. Provides programs and services for spiritual healing utilizing Jewish texts and traditions, New York program information 212-580-0099.

Lambda Legal Defense and Education Fund, 666 Broadway, New York, NY 10012, 212-995-8585. Test-case litigation for gay and lesbian issues and for all people living with AIDS, education and information. Publish a manual on legal issues and AIDS.

The Lighthouse, 800 Second Avenue, New York, NY 10017, 212-808-0077, TDD: 212-808-5544, FAX: 212-808-0110. Counseling, education, training and resources for the newly blind. Extensive experience with blindness related to AIDS.

Los Angeles Shanti Foundation, 1616 N. La Brea, Los Angeles, CA 90029, (213) 962-8196—Shanti runs emotional support groups, bereavement groups, multiple loss groups and an extensive education program for women and men, including the PLUS Weekend (Positive Living for US) that teaches those who newly test positive about community resources and understanding the disease.

Louise Hay House, P.O. Box 6204, Carson, CA 90749, 310-605-0601. Books, audiotapes and videos on self-healing with meditation and visualization.

Manhattan Center for Living, 704 Broadway, 3rd Floor, New York, NY 10003, 212-533-3550. Meditation workshops, counseling, rebirthing, nutrition, bodywork.

Minority Task Force on AIDS, 127 West 127th Street, Room 422, New York, NY 10027, 212-864-4046. Wide range of services for people living with AIDS.

Mothers of AIDS Patients (MAP), c/o Ann Wright, UCSD Medical Center, Social Work Department, H918, 225 Dickenson Ave, San Diego, CA 92103, 619-543-5730.

Mother's Love Support Network, Mildred Pearson, Founder, P.O. Box 874, New York, NY 10116, 718-599-5078, 718-383-4402. Support for mothers and grandmothers of adult children, living or deceased, with AIDS

National AIDS Information Clearinghouse, P.O. Box 6003, Rockville, MD 20850, 800-458-5231.

National Gay/Lesbian Health Education Foundation, P.O. Box 65472, Washington, D.C. 20035, 202-797-3708. Advocacy. Publishes sourcebook on gay/lesbian health care.

National Leadership Coalition on AIDS, 202-429-0930, Promotes fair AIDS policies in the workplace.

New Jersey Women and AIDS Network (NJWAN), 5 Elm Row, #112, New Brunswick, NJ 08901, 908-846-4462. The first organization of support, education and advocacy for women living with AIDS.

New York City AIDS Library, N.Y.C. Department of Health, 212-788-4280.

The New York Open Center, Inc., 83 Spring Street, New York, NY 10012, 212-219-2527. This school offers all kinds of alternative courses and programs, and has a mail-order bookstore.

Northern Light Alternatives, 601 West 50th Street, 5th Floor, New York, NY 10019, 212-765-3202. Branches in numerous cities. Retreats including self-help, motivation and meditation for people living with AIDS.

Nutritionists in AIDS Care (NAIC), c/o The New York Dietetic Association, P.O. Box 871, Lenox Hill Station, New York, NY 10021, 212-439-8073. Nutritionists and dieticians offering nutritional counseling, and referrals for food resources

People With AIDS Coalition, 50 # West 17th Street, 7th Floor, New York, NY 10011, 212-647-1415, Hotline: 800-828-3280. Offers counseling and programs for people living with AIDS. There are branches throughout the U.S.

People with AIDS Coalition of New York: The Living Room, 222 West 11th Street, New York, NY 10014, 718-934-1758 Beverly Rotter. Support Group for mothers whose adult children have died from AIDS.

Pet Owners with AIDS/ARC Resource Services (POWARS), 212-744-0842. Complete pet care services for people living with AIDS.

Rural AIDS Network, 505-986-8337. Conferences, education, support services.

Senior Action in a Gay Environment (SAGE), 208 West 13th Street, New York, N.Y. 10011, 212-741-2247. AIDS prevention and education for senior centers and programs.

The Shanti Project, 525 Howard Street, San Francisco, CA 94105, 415-777-2273. Practical and emotional support for people living with AIDS and their loved ones.

We The People (Philadelphia), 215-545-6868. Counseling, housing referrals and advocacy.

The Wellness Center, 145 West 28th Street, 9th Floor, New York, NY 10001, 212-465-8062. Self-help and self-healing seminars, cleansing work and clonic and polarity sessions.

Whitman-Walker Clinic, Washington, D.C., 202-797-3500. Speakers, street outreach, information.

Women's AIDS Resource Network, 30 Third Avenue, Suite 212, Brooklyn, NY 11217, 718-596-6007. Crisis intervention, case management and outreach programs.

Women's Center and AIDS Project (WCAP) Women's Action Alliance, 370 Lexington Avenue, Room 603, New York, NY 10017, 212-532-8330. Publishes a resource list of educational materials on AIDS-related issues for women and families.

Books on Surviving AIDS

There are a lot of books available for people to use to find inspiration and ideas on "how to" survive AIDS. By the time you read this list, it will be obsolete, since new books are coming out daily. I would suggest going to the library or bookstores and checking out what they have. Focus on the books which combine both the medical materials and practical and specific guidance to help people living with AIDS take greater control over their own lives. A medical handbook might be good for doctors, but most that I have seen ignore the person and focus on a disease or symptoms. The following are books which I feel are of particular help and interest:

The AIDS Book: Creating a Positive Approach, Louise Hay, Hay House, Santa Monica, CA. 1988. If read carefully, this brilliant and helpful work can make real and meaningful differences in people's lives. Be careful: Louise doesn't accuse people of being at fault for their illness, she does say that the mind and the body are connected, and the body is telling us something we should listen to. Her issue is not blame—it's understanding, growth and inner peace.

AIDS: A Self-Care Manual, edited by Betty Clare Mofatt, Judith Spiegel, Steve Parrish and Michael Helquist, AIDS Project Los Angeles, CA. 1987. Dated, but still a useful guidebook covering all aspects of living with AIDS including legal, medical, communal and spiritual concerns.

AIDS Facts and Issues, edited by Victor Gong and Norman Rudnick, Rutgers University Press, New Brunswick, NJ. 1987. Comprehensive guide to problems surrounding AIDS. Includes studies by experts on tough issues—ethical , public health, legal, economic, spiritual, psychosocial, as well as basic information and resources.

AIDS, Macro-biotics and Natural Immunity, Michio Kushi, Martha Cottrell and Mark Mead, Japan Publications, NY. 1990. This tremendous volume is complete with everything you need to know (including recipes and personal accounts) about how a macrobiotic diet can help in survival.

Alive and Well: A Path for Living in Time of HIV, Peter Hendrickson, Irvington Publishers Inc.., NY. 1991. Lots of good information, especially when he gets into meditation and healing. I couldn't have said it better!

Beyond AIDS: A Journey into Healing, George Melton, Brotherhood Press, Beverly Hills, CA. 1988. This little pink book is amazing. George describes how he and his lover, Wil Garcia, left AIDS behind in their lives and found a way to live and be well. I thought this was fantasy and a great fairy tale when I read it, but the *Parade Magazine* (January 31, 1993) featured a story on "People Who Survive AIDS," and there was George Melton's face and story as proof that he has lasted from 1988's publication date until 1993—already a record! He should continue to live and be well.

The Caregiver's Journey: When You Love Someone With AIDS, Mel Pohl, M.D., Deniston Kay, Ph.D and Doug Toft, Hazeldon Books, New York. 1990. Practical information for caregivers, both lay and professional. Delineates stages of caregivers' journeys. Addresses issues of codependency, drug and alcohol abuse.

The Essential AIDS Fact Book, Paul Harding Douglas and Laura Pinsky, Pocket Books, NY. 1989. Comprehensive book on medical aspects of living with and preventing AIDS, including resource guide.

Healing AIDS Naturally, Laurence Badgley, Human Energy Press, Foster City, CA. 1987.

How to Find Information About AIDS, edited by Jeffrey Huber, Ph.D., Harington Park Press, NY. 1992. Really useful directory of where to find whatever you need, including organizations, foundations, audio-visual educational materials, electronic sources of information, grants.

Living in Hope: A 12-Step Approach for Persons at Risk or Infected with HIV, Cindy Mikluscak-Cooper, R.N. and Emmett E. Miller, M.D., Celestial Arts, Berkeley, CA. 1991. From the titles of the authors, I expected a medical approach, but this book is a brilliant, special application of the 12-step model to living with AIDS, with a lot of emphasis on the spiritual, self-help, mind/body approach. The Imagery Appendix is one which can be of tremendous value to people living with AIDS.

No Time to Wait: A Complete Guide to Treating, Managing and Living with HIV Infection, Nick Siano with Susan Lipsett, Bantam Books, NY. 1993. Wonderful, detailed explanation of the ways in which HIV works, discussion of medications and therapies including case studies, examination of alternate approaches, nutrition, mind/body connections.

Strategies for Survival: A Gay Health Manual for the Age of AIDS, Dr. Martin Delaney and Peter Goldblum, with Joseph Brewer, St. Martin's Press, NY. 1987. A somewhat dated workbook with a whole lot of good ideas which are timeless. Martin Delaney is the founding director of Project Inform, which supplies AIDS treatment information worldwide. This book should be required reading!

Surviving AIDS, Michael Callen, Harper Perennial, NY. 1991. May Michael be remembered for his heroism and leadership in the struggle to survive. This book is useful, insightful and brilliantly written.

Surviving With AIDS, C. Callaway and Catherine Whiten, Little Brown, Boston. 1991. Focuses on nutrition and survival.

Take These Broken Wings and Learn to Fly: The AIDS Support Book for Patients, Family and Friends, Steven D. Dietz and M. Jane Parker-Hicks, M.D., Harbinger House, Tucson, AZ. 1989. Good on psychological information, practical, offers hope.

When Someone You Know Has AIDS: A Practical Guide, Martelli, Peltz and Messina, Crown Publishers, NY. 1987. A little dated, but filled with practical ideas and insights. New edition is available.

Why I Survived AIDS, Niro Markoff Assistant, Simon and Schuster, New York, 1991. Practical, useful, filled with great suggestions for healing within.

You Can't Afford the Luxury of a Negative Thought, John-Roger and Peter McWilliams, Bantam Books, NY. 1991.

Self-Healing, Meditation and Prayer

AIDS and the Healer Within, Nick Bamforth, Amethyst Books, NY. 1993. Built around six Chakras, the book contains useful philosophy of meditation and self-healing and brilliant meditations and visualizations. This book does precisely what the cover says—guides us in the process of self-healing.

Creative Visualization, Shakti Gawain, New World Library, San Rafael, CA. 1978. Good visualizations, worth incorporating into your repertoire.

Guided Imagery, Larry Moen, both Volumes One and Two, United Stated Publishing, Naples, FL. 1992. The imagery and visualizations in these books are some of the best anywhere. Read them. Put the ones that are most meaningful onto tape, using your own voice. Enjoy!

Healing Visualizations: Creating Health Through Imagery, Gerald Epstein, M.D. Bantam Books, NY. 1989. Got a cold, dizziness, migraines, swelling? Dr. Epstein has the visualization which can help to cure the problem, alleviate the pain, or whatever you need. This book is a great resource for everyone interested in visualizing and actualizing healing.

Healing into Life and Death, Stephen Levine, Anchor Books, NY. 1987. Excellent explanation of "healing" and good technique for achieving healing. The meditations and visualizations are very complex and I have to admit, most of this book was over my head.

Jewish Meditation, Aryeh Kaplan, Schocken Books, NY. 1985. The introduction to Jewish meditation for anyone who thinks meditation is not a part of our tradition.

Inner Space, Aryeh Kaplan, Moznayim. 1990. Making room for that personal Jewish inner space? Once you find the space, add in the visualizations from all of the other sources.

The Power is Within You, Louise Hay, Hay House, Carson, CA. 1991. Focus on the Loving Yourself section, though the rest of the book is also worthwhile.

Peace, Love and Healing, Bernie Siegel, M.D. Walker, NY. 1990, and *Love, Medicine and Miracles*, Bernie Siegel, M.D., Harper-Collins, NY. 1990. Both books show clearly that the medical model which ignores the emotional/spiritual concerns of the patient is of little help. Bernie's books and meditation tapes are useful and inspiring, and should be required medical school texts. These are the books with which to start learning about our roles in our own healing.

Quantum Healing: Exploring the Frontiers of Mind/Body Medicine, Deepak Chopra, Bantam Books, NY. 1990. Fascinating reading. Check it out.

Trusting the Healing Within, Nick Bamforth, Amethyst Books, Woodstock, NY. 1989.

Working Inside Out, Margo Adair, Wingbow Press, Berkeley, CA. 1985. Step-by-step guide on meditation. Cassettes are also available for people who are HIV positive and worried. Write to: Tools for Change, Box 14141, San Francisco, CA 94114.

You Can Heal Your Life, Louise Hay, Hay House, Carson, CA. 1987. General thoughts on healing your body and soul. All of Louise's books are good and all give new insights, techniques and ideas for healing.

Inspiration

The Bible, particularly the Book of Psalms! Check out Psalms 4, 5, 6, 16, 20, 23, 25, 30, 38, 46, 103, 130. The list was provided by my teacher, Rabbi Bernard Zlotowitz. Any translation is okay but I recommend the Jewish Publication Society's modern translations of Psalms and the Bible.

A Course in Miracles, Foundation for Inner Peace, Tiburon, CA. 1992.

Head First: The Biology of Hope, Norman Cousins, Viking Penguin, NY. 1990.

Chicken Soup for the Soul: 101 Stories to Open the Heart and Rekindle the Spirit, Jack Canfield and Mark Hansen, Health Communications, Inc., Deerfield Beach, FL. 1993. With a name like this, how can you go wrong? Great stories and real food for thought.

The Color of Light: Meditations for All of Us Living With AIDS, Perry Tilleraas, Hazelden, Harper-Collins, NY. 1988. Each page is for one day. Each day includes a thought by a person whose life is touched by AIDS or another source, reflections and a positive affirmation. The book has tremendous power to change lives and raise spirits.

Heart Thoughts: A Treasury of Inner Wisdom, Louise Hay, Hay House, Carson, CA. 1990. Wonderful meditations and affirmations.

I Am Not a Victim: One Man's Triumph Over Fear and AIDS, Louie Nassaney with Glenn Kolb, Hay House, Carson, CA. 1990. Tells the story of Louie's life after diagnosis, how he survives using Louise Hay's approach. AIDS is written 'aids" throughout, to diminish its power—it shouldn't be in all caps. Just that thought makes this book worth considering.

Living in the Light, Shakti Gawain, New World Library, San Rafael, CA. 1987.

Love is Letting Go of Fear, Gerald Jampolsky, M.D., Celestial Arts, Berkeley, CA. 1979. Based on *A Course in Miracles*, this book focuses on personal transformation and has lots of great exercises.

100 Blessings Every Day, Rabbi Kerry Olitzky, Jewish Lights Publishing, Woodstock, VT. 1993. Written for people in 12-Step programs and recovery, the book contains meditations for each day of the Hebrew calendar, including a reading from traditional Jewish sources, thoughts and reflections and a suggestion for "growth and renewal." Many people living with AIDS also have experienced and needed to recover from alcoholism, drug abuse, chemical dependence, and codependency in relationships. This book is particularly useful for people familiar with 12-Step programs, but everyone else can also benefit from its daily use.

Out of the Darkness into the Light: A Journey of Inner Healing, Gerald Jampolsky, M.D., Bantam Books, NY. 1989. Tells the story of the author's personal transformation from alcoholism to inner healing and peace. Contains some great stories, prayers and readings.

Renewed Each Day: Daily Twelve Step Recovery Meditations Based on the Bible, Rabbi Kerry Olitzky and Aaron Z., Jewish Lights Publishing, Woodstock, VT. Built on the weekly Torah portion, each daily meditation is connected with the Torah portion, Jewish insight and sources. This book is a wonderful resource.

Serenity, Paul Reed, Celestial Art, Berkeley, CA. 1990. Paul Reed is a noted author of gay literature, and this book is a beautiful account of his personal reflections and techniques for coping with AIDS. A meaningful book which can help bring inspirations and serenity to people living with AIDS and the people who love them.

A Treasury of Comfort, edited by Rabbi Sidney Greenberg, Wilshire Book Company, N. Hollywood, CA. 1954. Written as a source of consolation and hope for people who are in mourning, this book has some wonderful readings which are helpful and inspiring for a much wider range of people, including people facing their own deaths and seeking comfort and hope. The resources included here can be tremendously helpful for people who know that their time in this world is very short, as well as to their loved ones in accepting and easing the transition to *Olam HaBah* (the next world).

Twice Blessed: On Being Lesbian, Gay, and Jewish, edited by Christie Balka and Andy Rose, Beacon Press, Boston. 1989. The best book on the issue of being twice blessed. If you have issues of how to deal with people who are gay and living with AIDS, read this book.

Walking Humbly with God, The Life and Writings of Rabbi Hershel Jonah Matt, edited by Daniel Matt, KTAV Publishing, Hoboken, NJ. 1993. Read the articles on homosexuality, and the *kavvanot* and prayers.

When All You've Ever Wanted Isn't Enough, Rabbi Harold Kushner, Simon & Schuster, 1986. What's missing in your life? Channel your energies into the "right" directions.

When Bad Things Happen to Good People, Rabbi Harold Kushner, Avon Books, NY. 1983. Since the time of Job, we have been struggling to understand this question. Rabbi Kushner's work helps all of us to forget about the question "why me?" and focus on our energies in the positive direction of "now what do I do?"

Thinking About Olam HaBah (the world to come)

Let's face it, all of us die. People living with AIDS, and people who work with people living with AIDS, have to face the issues of death, dying, mourning, grief and remembering. Buddies often replace family members who either will not or cannot walk this path with people living with AIDS, and the loss and grief a buddy feels are intense and real. The following books can be helpful in preparing for the death of a loved one, and in working through the grief.

After you Say Goodbye: When Someone You Love Dies of AIDS, Froman, Chronicle Books, San Francisco, CA. 1992.

Beyond Grief, Carol Staudacher, New Harbinger Publications, Oakland, CA. 1987.

Eschatology-The Doctrine of a Future Life in Israel, Judaism and Christianity, R.H. Charles, Schocken Books, NY. 1963.

Jewish Attitudes Toward the Afterlife, Simcha Paull Rafael, Ph.D., Jason Aronson, Northvale, NJ forthcoming. I have had the pleasure of meeting Simcha and hearing a lecture on the afterlife and Judaism. For information about his bereavement services and death education classes, call 215-848-0358.

A Jewish Book of Comfort, Alan A. Kay, Jason Aronson, NJ. 1993. Alan is a colleague of mine at The Academy for Jewish Religion and a respected professor of English. This book is the result of his personal struggle with grief at the death of his father and contains over 175 short essays, fiction, stories, poems, insights and readings from traditional Jewish sources.

The Jewish Mourner's Handbook, edited by William Cutter, Behrman House, West Orange, N.J. 1992. Useful, basic-level information about funerals and mourning.

The Jewish Way in Death and Mourning, Maurice Lamm, Jonathan David Publishing., NY. 1969. Comprehensive going from the moment of death through the funeral, mourning, post mourning, and "the world beyond the grave."

Judaism and Immortality, Levi Olan, UAHC, New York. 1971.

Life After Life, Raymond Moody, Jr., M.D. Bantam Books, NY. 1976. Reflections on near-death experiences of people who have died and been revived.

A Minyan of Comfort, compiled and edited by Rabbi Sidney Greenberg and Rabbi Jonathan Levine, published by Prayer Book Press, Media Judaica, Bridgeport, CT. 1991. The best prayer book for use during *shiva*. The prayers and readings are meaningful; the right thoughts at the right time.

Moses Maimonides' Treatise on Resurrection, translated and edited by Fred Rosner, Ktav Publishing, NY. 1983.

Mourning and Mitzvah, Anne Brener, Jewish Lights Publishing, VT. 1993. The book is extremely useful for helping people to understand Jewish traditions and rituals around death and to find personal meanings in them. The thoughts and meditations are incredible!

On Death and Dying, Elizabeth Kubler-Ross, MacMillan, NY. 1969. The definitive work on the process of coming to terms with our own mortality and with grieving a loss.

Open Hands: A Jewish guide on Dying, Death and Bereavement, Rami Shapiro, Temple Beth Or, Miami, FL. 1986.

So That Your Values Live on: Ethical Wills and How to Prepare Them, edited and annotated by Jack Reimer and Nathaniel Stampfer, Jewish Lights Publishing, VT. 1991. There's more to life and death than who gets the stereo, and this book demonstrates that we leave much more than things behind. People living with AIDS might want to consider the other kinds of "wills." The book includes interesting excerpts of the ethical wills of a wide variety of people, famous and ordinary.

The Way of Splendor—Jewish Mysticism and Modern Psychology, Edward Hoffman, Shambhala Publications, Boulder, CO. 1981. Chapter on "Life and Death—the Immortal Soul." Well worth reading the whole book.

What Happens After I Die: Jewish Views of Life After Death, Rifat Sonsino and Daniel Syme, UAHC Press, NY. 1989. The book has two parts: Classic Jewish Positions and Contemporary Thinkers, including some really interesting essays by representatives of different movements. Maybe I was expecting too much in looking for the definitive and authoritative answer to the title question.

Who Dies? an Investigation of Conscious Living and Conscious Dying, Stephen Levine, Anchor Books, NY. 1982. When you're living with a chronic, potentially fatal disease or are the caretaker for someone who is, this book can provide meaningful guidance and insights. The chapter "Healing/Dying—The Great Balancing Act" is one to focus on.

Willow Baskets, Colored Glasses: A Friend's Guide to Comforting Mourners, Rami Shapiro, Temple Beth Or, Miami, FL. 1988.

*P*ermissions

Every effort has been made to ascertain the owners of copyrights for the selections used in this volume, and to obtain permission to reprint copyrighted passages. Alef Design Group will be pleased, in subsequent editions, to correct any inadvertent errors or omissions that may be pointed out.